Meaning-Centered Group Psychotherapy for Patients with Advanced Cancer

Meaning-Centered Group Psychotherapy for Patients with Advanced Cancer

A Treatment Manual

WILLIAM S. BREITBART, MD

Interim Chairman
Chief, Psychiatry Service, Department of Psychiatry and Behavioral Sciences
Attending Psychiatrist, Pain & Palliative Care Service, Department of Neurology
Memorial Sloan-Kettering Cancer Center
Professor of Clinical Psychiatry, Department of Psychiatry
Weill Medical College of Cornell University
New York, New York

SHANNON R. POPPITO, PHD

Clinical Psychologist/Behavioral Health Consultant
Behavioral Health Optimization Program
Los Angeles Air Force Base
61st Medical Squadron
Los Angeles, California

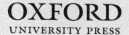

OXFORD
UNIVERSITY PRESS

OXFORD

UNIVERSITY PRESS

Oxford University Press is a department of the University of
Oxford. It furthers the University's objective of excellence in research,
scholarship, and education by publishing worldwide.

Oxford   New York
Auckland   Cape Town   Dar es Salaam   Hong Kong   Karachi
Kuala Lumpur   Madrid   Melbourne   Mexico City   Nairobi
New Delhi   Shanghai   Taipei   Toronto

With offices in
Argentina   Austria   Brazil   Chile   Czech Republic   France   Greece
Guatemala   Hungary   Italy   Japan   Poland   Portugal   Singapore
South Korea   Switzerland   Thailand   Turkey   Ukraine   Vietnam

Oxford is a registered trademark of Oxford University Press
in the UK and certain other countries.

Published in the United States of America by
Oxford University Press
198 Madison Avenue, New York, NY 10016

Library of Congress Cataloging-in-Publication Data
Breitbart, William, 1951- author.
Meaning-centered group psychotherapy for patients with advanced cancer : a treatment manual / William S. Breitbart,
Shannon R. Poppito.
p. ; cm.
Includes bibliographical references and index.
ISBN 978–0–19–983725–0 (alk. paper) — ISBN 978–0–19–938067–1 (alk. paper)
I. Poppito, Shannon R., author. II. Title.
[DNLM: 1. Neoplasms—psychology. 2. Psychotherapy, Group—methods. 3. Depression--therapy. 4. Quality of Life.
5. Terminally Ill—psychology. QZ 200]
RC271.M4
616.99'40651—dc23
2013047207

9 8 7 6 5 4 3 2 1
Printed in the United States of America
on acid-free paper

But if there is meaning,
it is unconditional meaning,
and neither suffering nor dying
can detract from it.
What our patients need is
an unconditional faith
in this unconditional meaning.

Viktor Frankl, *The Will to Meaning* (1969, p. 156)

The image on the title page is a carving that was created by a meaning-centered psychotherapy study patient for his final "Legacy Project." It depicts his past, present, and future legacy intertwined within the symbol of his Irish heritage and bound together by "eternal love."

Contents

Acknowledgments

We are indebted to our families for their love and support, and remember those precious to us, both family and patients, who have died during the period of time we conducted the work reflected in this text.

We are indebted to our colleagues at Memorial Sloan-Kettering who played central roles in the development and conduct of trials of both meaning-centered psychotherapy (MCP) formats. Special thanks go to Mindy Greenstein, Hayley Pessin, Barry Rosenfeld, Wendy Lichtenthal, Allison Applebaum, and our many research collaborators, research assistants, interventionists, pre- and postdoctoral fellows, and research managers and coordinators.

We thank the National Institutes of Health, the National Cancer Institute, the National Center for Complementary and Alternative Medicine, the Fetzer Institute, and the Kohlberg Foundation, who provided funding for MCP clinical trials research.

Finally, our gratitude to the hundreds of patients who participated in the clinical trials of MCP, and their devoted families and caregivers. While most of the patients who participated in the clinical trials of MCP are no longer with us, their legacies are alive and affect the course and meaning of our lives in profound ways.

There is but one truly serious philosophical problem, and that is suicide. Judging whether life is or is not worth living amounts to answering the fundamental question of philosophy.. . . . I therefore conclude that the meaning of life is the most urgent of questions.

Albert Camus, *Myth of Sisyphus* (1955, pp. 3–4)

If you have opened this treatment manual and are reading this preface, you are likely a clinician or researcher who works with cancer patients (and perhaps specifically with advanced cancer and palliative care populations) and who has come to understand, either through repeated clinical experience or our contributions to the clinical research literature, the importance of helping patients sustain a sense of meaning, particularly in the last months of life as they confront death. Like Camus, you have concluded that "meaning of life is the most urgent of questions." Perhaps it is more accurate to say that you have come to learn, as our research group has, that the ability to sustain or enhance meaning in advanced cancer patients helps them maintain a sense of hope and purpose, improve quality of life and reduce symptom distress, and diminish despair. You have also learned that central to the concept of "care" for advanced cancer patients is an approach to care that promotes the belief that "the possibility of creating or experiencing meaning exists until the last moment of life."

It has been close to a decade since our research group at Memorial Sloan-Kettering found its way to understanding the clinical and existential importance of meaning and the preservation of meaning as a concept central to a psychotherapeutic intervention for patients with advanced cancer who, in fact, were facing death. We came to call this intervention "Meaning-Centered Psychotherapy" (MCP) and first developed, tested, and ultimately proved efficacious in randomized controlled trials, a group format of MCP we called "Meaning-Centered

Group Psychotherapy" (MCGP). MCGP is an eight-week intervention, composed of didactics and experiential exercises. It is designed to help advanced cancer patients understand the importance and relevance of sustaining, reconnecting with, and creating meaning in their lives through common and reliable sources of meaning that may serve as resources of meaning that help to diminish despair near the end of life.

In this preface to *Meaning-Centered Group Psychotherapy for Patients with Advanced Cancer*, we briefly present the scientific rationale for MCGP as an effective intervention for patients with advanced cancer. The manual itself is very detailed and we trust will be a step-by-step guide for clinicians and researchers to use in applying the intervention in clinical settings, or to conduct replication studies, or develop adaptations off the intervention for local cultures and languages. It is recommended that the reader refer to the forthcoming Oxford University Press textbook *Meaning-Centered Psychotherapy for Cancer*, by Drs. Breitbart and Poppito, for detailed descriptions of therapeutic techniques utilizing transcripted examples of therapeutic encounters. In addition, the reader may be interested in the treatment manual for *Individual Meaning-CenteredPsychotherapy for Patients with Advanced Cancer* also published by Oxford University Press and authored by Drs. Breitbart and Poppito.

Developing Meaning-Centered Group Psychotherapy

Like many clinical interventions in the fields of psycho-oncology and palliative care, MCP, and MCGP in particular, arose from a need to deal with a challenging clinical problem—a problem for which no effective intervention was, as yet, available. In fact, it was through the fortunate collision of encountering a clinical problem in the context of being inspired by the works of pioneers in existential philosophy and psychiatry that MCP was conceived, developed, tested, and ultimately demonstrated to be an effective intervention in a group format. The clinical problem was despair, hopelessness, and desire for hastened death in advanced cancer patients who were in fact not suffering from a clinical depression (Breitbart et al., 2000), but rather confronting an existential crisis of loss of meaning, value, and purpose, in the face of a terminal prognosis. While our group ultimately demonstrated that desire for hastened death in the presence of a clinical depression could be reversed with adequate antidepressant therapy (Breitbart et al., 2010), no effective intervention was available for loss of meaning and hopelessness in the absence of clinical depression. Inspired primarily by the works of Viktor Frankl (1955, 1959, 1969, 1975) and further informed by the contributions of Irvin Yalom (1980) our research group adapted Frankl's concepts of the importance of meaning in human existence (and his "logotherapy"), and initially created a meaning-centered intervention in a group format (MCGP), intended primarily for advanced cancer patients. The goal of the intervention was to diminish despair, demoralization, hopelessness, and desire for hastened death by sustaining or enhancing a sense of meaning, even in the face of death. While MCP relies heavily on Frankl's concepts of meaning and sources of meaning as resources to reconnect with meaning in the midst of suffering, MCP also incorporates important and fundamental existential concepts and concerns that do not directly focus on meaning, but are clearly related to the search for, connection with, and creation of meaning.

The Importance of Meaning and Spiritual and Existential Well-Being in Coping with Cancer

There is extensive evidence that demonstrates the significance of meaning and existential or spiritual well-being for patients with advanced cancer. Singer and colleagues found that "achieving a sense of spiritual peace" was a domain of end-of-life care that was most important from the patients' perspective (Singer, Martin, & Kelner, 1999). Moadel and colleagues surveyed 248 cancer patients and asked them what their most important needs were (Moadel et al., 1999). 51% said they needed help overcoming fears, while 41% needed help finding hope, 40% needed help finding meaning in life, 43% needed help finding peace of mind, and 39% needed help finding spiritual resources. In a sample of 162 Japanese hospice inpatients, psychological distress was related to meaninglessness in 37%, hopelessness in 37%, and loss of social role and feeling irrelevant in 28% (Morita, Tsunoda, Inoue, & Chihara, 2000). In a survey conducted by Meier and colleagues of the reasons for patient requests for assisted suicide, physicians reported that "loss of meaning in life" accounted for 47% of the requests (Meier et al., 1998). Clearly, from patient and physician perspectives alike, issues of spirituality are essential elements of quality end-of-life care. Brady and colleagues found that cancer patients who reported a high degree of meaning in their lives were able to report higher satisfaction with their quality of life and to tolerate severe physical symptoms better than patients who reported lower levels of meaning/peace (Brady et al., 1999). Our research group (Breitbart et al., 2000; Nelson, Rosenfeld, Breitbart, & Galietta, 2002) has demonstrated a central role for spiritual well-being, and meaning in particular, as a buffering agent, protecting against depression, hopelessness, and desire for hastened death among terminally ill cancer patients. McClain and colleagues found that the meaning component of spiritual well-being was significantly associated with end-of-life despair (as defined by hopelessness, desire for hastened death, and suicidal ideation), even after controlling for the influence of depression (McClain, Rosenfeld, & Breitbart, 2003). Yanez and colleagues similarly found that increases in meaning/peace in breast cancer survivors significantly predicted better mental health and lower distress, whereas increases in faith did not (Yanez et al., 2009).

This research highlights the role of meaning as a buffer against depression, hopelessness, suicidal ideation, and desire for hastened death, and is significant in the face of what we know about the consequences of depression and hopelessness in cancer patients. Depression, hopelessness, and loss of meaning are associated with poorer survival (Watson et al., 1999) and higher rates of suicide, suicidal ideation, hopelessness, and desire for hastened death (Breitbart & Rosenfeld, 1999; Breitbart et al., 2000; Chochinov et al., 1994, 1995; Kissane et al., 1997).

Additionally, hopelessness and loss of meaning have been shown to be independent of depression as predictors of desire for death, and are as influential on desire for death as depression (Breitbart et al., 2000). Therefore, there was a critical need for the development of psychosocial interventions for advanced cancer patients that addresses loss of meaning as a mechanism for improving psychosocial outcomes (e.g., quality of life, depression, anxiety, hopelessness, desire for death, and end-of-life despair).

Also important to the theoretical conceptual model of MCP is Park and Folkman's (1997) concept of a form of "meaning-focused coping."

They describe meaning in terms of reevaluating an event and the extent to which one has "made sense of" or "found meaning" in an event (Andrykowski, Brady, & Hunt, 1993; Folkman, 1997; Frankl 1955, 1959, 1969, 1975; Taylor, 1983, 1993).

Unlike Park and Folkman's conceptualization of meaning as global or situational, Frankl viewed meaning as a state; individuals can move from feeling demoralized and as if their lives hold no value (see Kissane et al., 1997), to recognizing their personal sense of meaning and purpose, which allows them to value even more intensely the time remaining. Conceptualizing meaning as a state subject to change suggests its potential responsiveness to intervention. Frankl also viewed suffering as a potential springboard, both for having a need for meaning and for finding it (Frankl, 1955, 1959). Hence, the diagnosis of a terminal illness may be seen as a crisis in the fullest sense of the word—an experience of distress or even despair that may in itself offer an opportunity for growth and meaning. Either one has a loss of sense of meaning and purpose in life, or one has a sustained or even heightened sense of meaning, purpose, and peace, which allows one to value more profoundly the time remaining and positively appraise events.

Drawing from these principles, MCGP helps to enhance patients' sense of meaning by helping them to understand and capitalize on the various sources of meaning in their lives. Enhanced meaning is conceptualized as the catalyst for improved psychosocial outcomes, such as improved quality of life, reduced psychological distress, and reduced despair. Specifically, meaning is viewed as both an intermediary outcome and a mediator of changes in these important psychosocial outcomes.

Concepts Central to Existential Philosophy and Psychology

Underlying the development and delivery of MCP and MCGP are concepts central to existential philosophy, psychology, and psychiatry, developed by such pioneers as Kierkegaard, Nietzsche, Heidegger, Sartre, Camus, and Yalom (Camus, 1955; Heidegger, 1996; Kierkegaard, Hong, & Hong, 1983; Nietzsche, 1986; Sartre, 1984; Yalom, 1980).

While concerns relating to meaning and meaninglessness are central to existential philosophy and psychology, MCP and MCGP have benefited from the incorporation of a number of important existential concepts that do not directly involve meaning, but are interrelated and serve as a critical framework for conducting the psychotherapeutic work of MCP. Therefore, although the emphasis of MCP is on meaning and sources of meaning, clearly much of the psychotherapeutic work is richer when therapists are well grounded in the basic conceptual framework and theories of existential philosophy and psychotherapy. Important existential concepts that are utilized and incorporated into the theoretical framework of MCP include: freedom, responsibility, choice, creativity, identity, authenticity, engagement, existential guilt, care, transcendence, transformation, direction, being unto death, being and temporality, and existential isolation. These existential concepts inform the intervention and are utilized primarily to reinforce the goals of MCP related to the search for, connection with, and creation of meaning.

Overview of Evidence on Efficacy of Meaning-Centered Group Psychotherapy (MCGP)

Prior to the development of MCGP, few interventions specifically focused on existential or spiritual domains in treatment, or measured the impact of treatment on such outcomes, particularly in patients with advanced cancer. Early research by Yalom, Spiegel, and colleagues demonstrated that a one-year supportive group psychotherapy that included a focus on existential issues decreased psychological distress and improved quality of life (Spiegel, Bloom, & Yalom, 1981; Spiegel & Yalom, 1978; Yalom & Greaves, 1977). More recent studies have described short-term interventions that included a spiritual or existential component, including individually based approaches (Chochinov et al., 2011; Kissane et al., 2003; Lee et al., 2006). However, the results of these studies are inconsistent in terms of their effects on psychological outcomes such as depression, anxiety, and desire for death. More importantly, specific aspects of spiritual well-being and meaning were not consistently targeted as outcomes. Thus, despite the seeming importance of enhancing one's sense of meaning and purpose, few clinical interventions have been developed that attempt to address this critical issue. Meaning-centered group psychotherapy was developed in response to the need for interventions that focused on enhancing spiritual well-being.

A randomized controlled trial of MCGP (Breitbart et al., 2010) demonstrated the efficacy of this intervention in improving spiritual well-being and a sense of meaning, as well as in decreasing anxiety, hopelessness, and desire for death. Ninety patients received either eight sessions of MCGP or supportive group psychotherapy (SGP). Fifty-five patients completed the eight-week intervention, and thirty-eight of these patients completed a follow-up assessment two months later (attrition between the two posttreatment assessments was largely due to patient death or physical deterioration). Outcome assessments included measures of spiritual well-being, meaning, hopelessness, desire for death, optimism/pessimism, anxiety, depression, and overall quality of life.

Results of this study demonstrated significantly greater benefits from MCGP compared to SGP, particularly in enhancing spiritual well-being and a sense of meaning. Treatment effects for MCGP appeared even stronger two months after treatment ended, suggesting that benefits not only persist, but may grow after treatment has been completed. Patients who participated in SGP failed to demonstrate any such improvements, either post treatment or at the two month follow-up assessment.

This study provides support for the effectiveness of MCGP as a novel intervention for improving spiritual well-being, a sense of meaning, and psychological functioning in patients with advanced cancer. Large treatment effects emerged after the short-term intervention, and these benefits appeared to increase even in the weeks after treatment ended. Although preliminary, MCGP appears to be a promising intervention for the enhancement of quality of life for patients at the end of life. A five-year RO1-funded larger randomized controlled trial of MCGP has just been completed, and preliminary analyses further solidify the evidence base supporting the efficacy of MCGP.

Future Directions

MCGP has been demonstrated to be an effective intervention for patients with advanced cancer. Our group at Memorial Sloan-Kettering Cancer Center has recognized the importance of interventions aimed at enhancing meaning. We developed a more flexible individual format of MCP, "Individual Meaning-Centered Psychotherapy " (IMCP).

IMCP has proved to be equally effective as MCGP, but allows for more flexibility in time and place (e.g., office, bedside, or chemo suite) for scheduling sessions, and has reduced attrition and enhanced rates of intervention completers (Breitbart et al., 2012). A pilot randomized controlled trial of IMCP demonstrated that IMCP significantly improved patients' spiritual well-being, sense of meaning, quality of life, and symptom-related distress (Breitbart et al., 2012). We are currently adapting and testing MCP for other cancer populations, (e.g., breast cancer survivors, bereaved parents, informal cancer caregivers, adolescents and young adults with cancer) as well as for oncology care providers (Fillion et al., 2009). Replication studies of MCGP are being conducted in Italy, Israel, and Spain. Cultural and linguistic adaptations of MCGP are being conducted by our group for Chinese and Hispanic populations. Investigators in the Netherlands have adapted MCGP for Dutch cancer survivors.

Summary

MCGP represents the group format of MCP, developed by Breitbart and colleagues in the Department of Psychiatry and Behavioral Sciences, Memorial Sloan-Kettering Cancer Center. MCGP is a novel and unique intervention demonstrated to be effective in enhancing meaning and diminishing despair in advanced cancer patients. MCGP has great promise as an intervention that can be utilized in the palliative care setting, as well as in the acute cancer treatment setting for advanced cancer patients.

References

Andrykowski, M.A., Brady, M.J., & Hunt, J.W. (1993). Positive psychosocial adjustment in potential bone marrow transplant recipients: cancer as a psychosocial transition. *Psycho-Oncology, 2*, 261–276.

Brady, M.J., Peterman, A.H., Fitchett, G., Mo, M., & Cella, D. (1999). A case of including spirituality in quality of life measurement in oncology. *Psycho-Oncology, 8*, 417–428.

Breitbart, W., & Rosenfeld, B. (1999). Physician-assisted suicide: the influence of psychosocial issues. *Cancer Control, 6*, 146–161.

Breitbart, W., Rosenfeld, B., Pessin, H., Kaim, M., Funesti-Esch, J., Galietta, M., Nelson, C.J., & Brescia, R. (2000). Depression, hopelessness, and desire for hastened death in terminally ill patients with cancer. *Journal of the American Medical Association, 284,* 2907–2811.

Breitbart, W., Rosenfeld, B., Gibson, C., Kramer, M., Li, Y., Tomarken, A., Nelson, C., et al. (2010). Impact of treatment for depression on desire for hastened death in patients with advanced cancer. *Psychosomatics, 51,* 98–105.

Breitbart, W., Rosenfeld, B., Gibson, C., Pessin, H., Poppito, S., Nelson, C., Tomarken, A., et al. (2010). Meaning-centered group psychotherapy for patients with advanced cancer: a randomized controlled trial. *Psycho-Ongology, 19,* 21–28.

Breitbart, W., Poppito, S., Rosenfeld, B., Vickers, A.J., Li, Y., Abbey, J., Olden, M., et al. (2012). Pilot randomized controlled trial of individual meaning-centered psychotherapy for patients with advanced cancer. *Journal of Clinical Oncology, 30,* 1304–1309.

Camus, A. (1955). *The Myth of Sisyphus and Other Essays.* Knopf, New York.

Chochinov, H.M., Kristjanson, L.J., Breitbart, W., McClement, S., Hack, T.F., Hassard, T., & Harlos, M. (2011). Effect of dignity therapy on distress and end-of-life experience in terminally ill patients: a randomized controlled trial. *Lancet Oncology, 12*(8), 753–762.

Chochinov, H.M., Wilson, K.G., Enns, M., & Lander, S. (1994). Prevalence of depression in the terminally ill: effects of diagnostic criteria and symptom threshold judgments. *American Journal of Psychiatry, 51,* 537–540.

Chochinov, H.M., Wilson, K.G., Enns, M., Mowchun, N., Lander, S., Levitt, M., & Clinch, J.J. (1995). Desire for death in the terminally ill. *American Journal of Psychiatry, 152,* 1185–1191.

Fillion, L., Duval, S., Dumont, S., Gagnon, P., Tremblay, I., Bairati, I., & Breitbart, W. (2009). Impact of a meaning-centered intervention on job satisfaction and on quality of life among palliative care nurses. *Psycho-Oncology, 12,* 1300–1301.

Folkman, S. (1997). Positive psychological states and coping with severe stress. *Social Science and Medicine, 45,* 1207–1221.

Frankl, V.F. (1955/1986). *The Doctor and the Soul.* Random House, New York.

Frankl, V.F. (1959/1992). *Man's Search for Meaning,* Fourth Edition. Beacon Press, Boston.

Frankl, V.F. (1969/1988). *The Will to Meaning: Foundations and Applications of Logotherapy, Expanded Edition.* Penguin Books, New York.

Frankl, V.F. (1975/1997). *Man's Search for Ultimate Meaning.* Plenum Press, New York.

Heidegger, M. (1996). *Being and Time.* Translated by Joan Stambaugh. State University of New York Press, Albany.

Kierkegard, S., Hong, H., & Hong, E. (1983). *Fear and Trembling/Repetition.* Princeton University Press, Princeton, NJ.

Kissane, D., Block, S., Miach, P., Clarke, D.M., Ikin, J., Love, A., et al. (1997). Cognitive existential group therapy for patients with primary breast cancer—techniques and themes. *Psycho-Oncology, 6,* 25–33.

Kissane, D.W., Bloch, S., Smith, G.C., Miach, P., Clarke, D.M., Ikin, J., Love, A., et al. (2003). Cognitive existential group psychotherapy for women with primary breast cancer: a randomised controlled trial. *Psycho-Oncology, 12,* 532–546.

Lee, V., Cohen, S.R., Edgar, L., et al. (2006). Meaning-making and psychological adjustment to cancer: development of an intervention and pilot results. *Oncology Nursing Forum, 33,* 291–302.

McClain, C., Rosenfeld, B., & Breitbart, W. (2003). The influence of spirituality on end-of-life despair among terminally ill cancer patients. *Lancet, 361,* 1603–1607.

Meier, D.E., Emmons, C.A., Wallerstein, S., Quill, T., Morrison, R.S., & Cassel, C.K. (1998). A national survey of physician-assisted suicide and euthanasia in the United States. *New England Journal of Medicine, 338,* 1193–1201.

Moadel, A., Morgan, C., Fatone, A., Grennan, J., Carter, J., Laruffa, G., Skummy, A., & Dutcher, J. (1999). Seeking meaning and hope: self-reported spiritual and existential needs among an ethnically diverse cancer patient population. *Psycho-Oncology, 8,* 1428–1431.

Morita, T., Tsunoda, J., Inoue, S., & Chihara, S. (2000). An exploratory factor analysis of existential suffering in Japanese terminally ill cancer patients. *Psycho-Oncology, 9,* 164–168.

Nietzsche, F. (1986). *Human, All Too Human: A Book for Free Spirits.* Translated by R.J. Hollingdale. Cambridge University Press, Cambridge, UK.

Nelson, C., Rosenfeld, B., Breitbart, W., & Galietta, M. (2002). Spirituality, depression and religion in the terminally ill. *Psychosomatics, 43,* 213–220.

Park, C., & Folkman, S. (1997). Meaning in the context of stress and coping. *Review of General Psychology, 1,* 115–144.

Sartre, J.P. (1984). *Being and Nothingness.* Citadel Press, New York.

Singer, P.A., Martin, D.K., & Kelner, M. (1999). Quality end-of-life care: patients' perspectives. *Journal of the American Medical Association, 281,* 163–168.

Spiegel, D., Bloom, J., & Yalom, I.D. (1981). Group support for patients with metastatic breast cancer. *Archives of General Psychiatry, 38,* 527–533.

Spiegel, D., & Yalom, I. (1978). A support group for dying patients. *International Journal of Group Psychotherapy, 28,* 233–245.

Taylor, E.J. (1993). Factors associated with meaning in life among people with recurrent cancer. *Oncology Nursing Forum, 20,* 1399–1405.

Taylor, S.E. (1983). Adjustment to threatening events: A theory of cognitive adaptation. *American Psychologist, 38,* 1161–1173.

Watson, M., Haviland, J.J., Greer, S., Davidson, J., & Bliss, J.M. (1999). Influence of psychological response on survival in breast cancer population-based cohort study. *Lancet, 354,* 1331–1336.

Yalom, I.D. (1980). *Existential Psychotherapy.* Basic Books, New York.

Yalom, I., & Greaves, C. (1977). Group therapy with the terminally ill. *American Journal of Psychiatry, 134,* 396–400.

Yanez, B., Edmondson, D., Stanton, A.L., Park, C.L., Kwan, L., Ganz, P.A., & Blank, T.O. (2009). Facets of spirituality as predictors of adjustment to cancer: Relative contributions of having faith and finding meaning. *Journal of Consulting and Clinical Psychology, 77,* 730–741.

Introduction

Meaning-Centered Group Psychotherapy Treatment
Overview for Therapists

General Guidelines for Group Therapists

Meaning-centered psychotherapy (MCP) for advanced cancer patients was developed and tested in randomized controlled trials by Breitbart and colleagues at Memorial Sloan-Kettering Cancer Center. Therapists using this manual are referred to the forthcoming Oxford University Press textbook, *Meaning-Centered Psychotherapy in Cancer*. Meaning-making is the defining characteristic of human beings as a species. Meaning-making has been addressed by many existential philosophers and psychotherapists, including Yalom, Park and Folkman, Kierkegard, Nietzsche, and Heidegger. This meaning-centered group psychotherapy intervention is influenced, to a large degree, by the work of the existential psychiatrist Viktor E. Frankl. It is therefore useful for group therapists as well as patient participants to have some familiarity with Frankl's work. *Man's Search for Meaning* is a good start; the first half of the book contains a particularly vivid account of key aspects of his philosophy. Other useful sources describing Frankl's concepts of the importance of "meaning" include his books *The Will to Meaning* and *The Doctor and the Soul.*

Co-facilitation Model, Training, Skills, and Experience

In the developmental phases of meaning centered group psychotherapy (MCGP), it had always been anticipated that a group consisting of six to eight patients would need to be led by two co-therapists or co-facilitators, and this has been the case in the two randomized controlled trials conducted of MCGP in advanced cancer populations. Logistically, it is useful to have such a co-therapist or co-facilitator model in order to keep the flow of each session on track in achieving the goals and tasks of each session, as well as sharing the burden of group leadership. In the randomized controlled trial of MCGP to date, group therapists have typically had master's level training, or higher, in psychology, psychiatry, social work, or mental health counseling. It is also helpful for therapists to have experience and basic skills in generic group psychotherapy. We have successfully used a model of co-facilitation in which a more senior therapist has been paired with a more junior and less experienced therapist. In such cases, we have utilized predoctoral psychology students as co-facilitators, and can imagine the potential use of nurses or chaplains in such co-facilitator roles.

While this manual, and the accompanying Oxford University Press textbook, should be sufficient for most clinicians to start to use MCGP in their practices, advanced training workshops in MCP are routinely conducted at the Annual World Congresses of the International Psycho-oncology Society (www.IPOS-Society.org), the Annual Scientific Meetings of the American Psychosocial Oncology Society (www.APOS-Society. org), and at Memorial Sloan-Kettering Cancer Center Department of Psychiatry and Behavioral Sciences (http://www.mskcc.org/research/ psychiatry-behavioral-sciences).

Patient Selection

MCGP was developed as an existential intervention to help sustain and/ or enhance meaning and spiritual well-being in advanced cancer patients with relatively limited prognosis (approximately six months to a year). The intervention was not developed to treat a specific DSM psychiatric disorder (e.g., major depressive disorder) but rather to address meta-diagnostic constructs such as "despair," "loss of spiritual well-being," and "demoralization," which are also often manifest in reports of poor quality of life, hopelessness, desire for hastened death, depressive and anxious symptoms, and loss of meaning and spiritual well-being. The randomized controlled trials of MCGP included patients with stage III or IV solid cancers who had limited prognosis but were expected to be ambulatory and well enough to attend eight weekly group sessions and to be alive two months post treatment in order to fill out follow-up outcome assessment measures. These selection criteria were picked for practical as well as research reasons. We included solid tumor cancer patients because there was a comparable staging system across all solid cancers. The course of treatment for solid cancers was also comparable across the board. We did include lymphoma patients, but excluded leukemia patients because of the often different course of treatment trajectory, and the lack of comparable staging system. Those of you using MCGP clinically with patients can be more flexible in your choice of patient selection based on cancer diagnosis. However, one should keep in mind the need to form treatment groups where patients can relate to the other members of the group as being "in the same boat" as them. In the MCGP trials, we chose not to require a threshold criterion of distress or loss of meaning for entry into the trials. This was a practical decision again. We felt this would hamper our ability to recruit sufficient patients. In later trials of individual meaning-centered psychotherapy, we required a score of 4 or greater on a 0–10 numerical rating scale of distress. We did this to assure that there would be room for improvement that could be demonstrated in our intervention trials. When used clinically, MCGP can enhance or sustain meaning and hope in patients who have a wide range of severity of distress or loss of meaning. We found that patients who had a good sense of meaning and spiritual well-being benefited from MCGP. We also found that patients in despair (e.g., significant loss of meaning, distress) benefited significantly and that the mixture of both types of patients in a group proved quite helpful in the group process. The real concern in patient selection is which patients to exclude. We excluded patients who had severe untreated depression, other psychiatric disorders, or cognitive impairment that would have made meaningful participation in the group process impossible. We did find that patients with limited education or mild cognitive deficits due to brain metastases (e.g., concrete thinking) were able to comprehend the concepts of MCGP and participate in the group process. Some patients were more visibly ill and weak than others, but this was also usually manageable. It was also interesting to note that despite the inclusion of only patients with stage III or IV solid cancers, there was in fact a broad range among group members as to prognostic awareness. It was not unusual for a patient with stage IV lung cancer to use denial as a coping method and to state "I expect to beat this cancer." Despite such pronouncements, these patients participated fully in all the exercises including the exercise on "what would be a good death." One patient, despite his pronouncement that "I expect to beat this cancer" had already planned out his funeral, including the guest list, the music, and the type of flowers he wanted. Diverse stages of prognostic awareness are thus to be expected, and are not limitations to running successful MCGP groups.

The Purpose of This Intervention

1. To affirm the possibility of the experience and creation of meaning, even in the face of advanced cancer and a potentially limited prognosis.

2. To aid participants in their discovery, reconnection, maintenance, and even enhancement of a sense of meaning in life during cancer illness.

3. To facilitate a greater understanding of sources of meaning that can be used as resources of meaning even after a diagnosis of cancer.

4. To promote a supportive environment among cancer patients faced with similar challenges at a particularly difficult time of their lives.

The Goal of This Intervention

The ultimate goal of this intervention is to optimize coping through an enhanced sense of meaning and purpose, to make the most of the time the group members have left, regardless of how long or how limited that time is. It is important to keep in mind that it is the individual group members' responsibility to use the group to discover the sources of meaning in their lives; they are perceived not as passive recipients of the group leaders' wisdom, but instead as active participants in the process. The intervention is intended to help broaden the scope of possible sources of meaning, and to promote the use of sources of meaning as resources for coping, through the combination of: (1) didactic teaching of the importance of meaning in human existence, the available sources of meaning in human life, and the need for meaning-making as a defining human characteristic, (2) experiential group exercises and homework to enhance learning and the incorporation of the importance of meaning and the utilization of the sources of meaning into patients' lives, and (3) open-ended discussion, which includes interpretive comments by group leaders to promote emotional expression and to facilitate patients' adoption of a meaning-focused perspective on coping.

How to Use the Manual

In the interest of minimizing repetition, the manual begins each session with a didactic discussion of the relevant principles. Group leaders should familiarize themselves thoroughly with the manual before convening groups. Though the didactic portion is written in script form, this is done in order to give leaders an idea of the flow of ideas in the session. It is not required or expected that these portions be read verbatim, though it is important that all relevant points be addressed. If necessary, you may keep notes on index cards, for example, and handouts should be made available for group members in case they would like to review the information themselves. Time should be allotted for each participant to complete exercises and combine them with discussion. The manual will indicate when specific handouts will be required. All handouts for patients are included in the appendices of this therapist manual. Additionally, it may be useful to have a whiteboard on hand, to highlight discussion points for group members.

While this intervention is brief, focused, and somewhat directive as compared with other group interventions, such as supportive-expressive group psychotherapy, there is some room for interpretive comments, especially in elucidating sources of meaning and goals and themes, that will arise. It is hoped that participants come away from the group with a set of tools for enabling them to continue the work begun here. Responsibility is a crucial issue, and it extends to group members' feeling responsible to themselves and each other in finding what is meaningful in their lives. This responsibility also includes finding worthwhile definitions of what constitutes meaningfulness in the first place, as will be explored in session one, and will lay the basis for much of what follows.

Each session in this manual includes the following: (1) a title page; (2) a session overview, which gives a brief summary of the components of each session and the tasks that need to be completed; (3) a discussion of the session goals and content; (4) a description of the didactic portion of each session; (5) a discussion of the experiential exercise or homework review that is completed in each session; and (6) a Therapist Adherence Checklist and Group Process note. The Therapist Adherence Checklist is the measure we utilize during our randomized controlled trials comparing MCGP with supportive group psychotherapy. This checklist can therefore be utilized in similar research studies undertaken by users of this manual who are engaging in replication studies or other comparative intervention studies. The Therapist Adherence Checklist identifies the key components of each MCGP session, so clinicians can also use these as a brief guide for the content to be covered in each session.

The Importance of Seeking Themes

It is also useful to note group themes when they seem to arise across individuals or across sessions. Expounding on these will help individual members to feel like a part of something larger than themselves even within the confines of the room—as they experience each other as having a communal mission. This may be made more explicit in later sessions, when the topic of feeling like a part of something greater will be elaborated more fully. As an example of how themes can be used to explore goals, one patient, who, in contemplating what he would like to do in his remaining time, began giving examples of various work activities, all of which involved children and were outside his reach given his physical condition. When this theme of children was highlighted, the patient began to describe his wish to repair his relationship with his own children before he died, and soon embarked on this goal. Before ending sessions, group leaders should give brief recaps of some of the themes that have come up. At the completion of each session, group leaders complete a brief note using the Therapist Adherence Checklist.

Attitudes Toward Suffering and Choosing One's Attitude, or Cognitive Reframing

One of the goals of the group is to help reframe the experience of patients from that of dying to that of living in the face of the threat of dying and to facilitate the ability to recognize future opportunities for meaningful experiences despite the limitations placed on them by their illness or treatment. In *The Will to Meaning*, Frankl describes his logotherapy as the "treatment of the patient's attitude toward his un-changeable fate" (p. 6), and to explore ways in which suffering can be experienced from a more positive perspective. He viewed the bearing of suffering as one potential way of realizing one's own values in the way that one takes up personal challenges. Much of what Frankl describes in his clinical work involves the attitude people take toward their suf-fering. Rather than focusing on their sense of pain or suffering, they are directed to focus outward toward goals to achieve, tasks to fulfill, and responsibilities toward others.

When cancer illness strips one of so many aspects of life that were pre-viously somewhat under one's control, and starts to impinge on one's "freedom," the last vestige of freedom is our ability to choose the atti-tude we take toward any limitation that causes suffering. Learning that we have "choices," particularly the freedom to choose one's attitude to-ward, or how one responds to, cancer-related limitations, is often the central lesson of MCP for many patients.

One example he offers is of an elderly widower who is despondent over his wife's recent death. This situation is ultimately reframed as one in which the widower has saved his wife the suffering that he is now enduring, giving his suffering a purpose in the larger scheme of things. Another example is Professor Morris Schwartz, the subject of the book *Tuesdays with Morrie*, who is stricken with ALS, but takes comfort from his ability to use his debilitating illness to teach his student important life lessons and who takes pride in approaching death with "dignity, courage, humor, composure" (Albom, 1997, p. 21).

Some suffering, however, is unavoidable, as we all face disappointments in life—painful losses or threat of death. The attitude taken toward these kinds of suffering, toward a fate that potentially cannot be changed, could refer to many different things. For example, Frankl described one fellow concentration camp inmate who hoped that his suffering might somehow spare his family. Other examples include being a role model in terms of how one copes with his or her suffering, or experiencing suf-fering as a catalyst for changing some aspect of one's life. In other words, sometimes people reframe their suffering (assuming they don't have the control to remove the source of that suffering) and explore what purposes it might be used to serve at this point in their lives. Suffering is not inherently necessary for finding meaning, but it is one possible avenue for it.

Meaningfulness, in this view, is not something that can be taken for granted but is instead something to achieve. It is through such achievements that one can feel a sense of fulfillment or transcendence or even a feeling of being a part of something greater than oneself. What we strive for in life is not necessarily happiness, which can be elusive, but a sense of fulfillment and contentment through which happiness may eventually ensue.

Therapist Care Tenor

> *What matters is never a technique per se,*
> *but rather the spirit in which the technique is used.*
>
> —Viktor Frankl, *The Will to Meaning* (1969, p. 29)

One difficulty with the approach of cognitive reframing (e.g., we have the freedom to choose our attitude or response to suffering), concerns the potential for the therapist to be experienced as authoritarian and patronizing, a criticism that has been leveled at Frankl himself (Yalom, 1980). Also, the group leaders should not be in a position of saying that suffering is necessary to experience meaning but, instead, that meaning can be experienced either despite or even through how one copes with (or more precisely how one "responds to") the *unavoidable limitations or* suffering that has been given to them by life.

It is important to highlight aspects of group members' *own experiences* that are consonant with a sense of meaningfulness rather than imposing one's own theories on them. An example of this occurred when a patient with end-stage cancer expressed concern that she not be a burden on her family. When she described having cared for loved ones during their illnesses in the past, the facilitator asked how it had felt to care for them. She said it had been very meaningful for her to be there for her loved ones and she was grateful for the opportunity to comfort them in their final days. When asked if she thought her family might feel similarly about caring for her, she responded that she had never thought to look at it that way.

Care must be taken not to have the facilitators simply impose a more positive spin on a participant's attitude, but rather, to explore *from the individual participant's perspective* the possibility of meaning. In the above example, the notion of burden was reframed as a gift in which the patient was giving someone else the opportunity to take care of her; but this reframing occurred within the context of exploring *her own* experience. It should be noted as well that the group itself provides members with a new goal, namely, to be in a position to help each other explore what is meaningful through empathy, compassion, and understanding.

Homework and Experiential Exercises in the Group

Each session in the manual contains experiential exercises that are meant to enhance the learning experience and help patients understand the concepts of MCP in a personal and profound way. After each session, patients are presented with homework assignments that are typically previews of the experiential exercises that they will participate in the following session. Many patients will review this homework and even prepare written responses to the stimulus questions that they will share during the group. It is not atypical (perhaps even more common than not) for patients to merely examine these homework assignments outside of session and contemplate their responses but not document them in writing. During each group session, we typically provide time for patients to write their responses to the stimulus questions of the experiential exercise prior to the sharing their responses with the group.

Concepts and Sources of Meaning

Introductions and Meaning

*Life holds meaning for each and every individual, and even more, it
retains this meaning literally to his last breath. And the [therapist] can
show his patient that life never ceases to have a meaning. To be sure,
he cannot show his patient what the meaning is, but he may well show
him that there is a meaning, and that life retains it: that it remains
meaningful, under any conditions. . . . Even the tragic and negative
aspects of life, such as unavoidable suffering, can be turned into a
human achievement by the attitude which a man adopts toward his
predicament . . . transforming despair into triumph.*

—Viktor Frankl, *The Will to Meaning* (1969, ix)

Session 1 Overview

1. INTRODUCTIONS—GROUP WELCOME
   • General Introductions
     • Group leader and member introductions
     • Intervention overview (e.g., treatment goals, logistics)
   • Introduction to Session 1
     • Goal #1: learn patients' cancer stories
     • Goal #2: Introduce concepts and sources of meaning

2. PATIENTS' CANCER STORIES

3. PATIENTS' DEFINITIONS OF MEANING

4. STUDY'S DEFINITIONS OF MEANING

5. EXPERIENTIAL EXERCISE MEANINGFUL MOMENTS

6. SESSION WRAP-UP
   • Brief summation of group session
   • Brief overview of next week's session—"Cancer and Meaning"

- Homework: read first chapter of Frankl's *Man's Search for Meaning*
- Reminder of following session (day/time)

Session Preparation

Co-facilitators should briefly meet ten to fifteen minutes before the session begins to prepare for the group. During this time, they should make sure they have the exercise and homework handouts available (and should ensure that the audiotape and/or video recorder are working properly if this is being done for research or training purposes). Handouts, exercises, and homework found at the end of this manual should be readied for distribution to group participants.

Session Goals

During this preparatory period, facilitators should reflect on and briefly discuss the topic and goals for this session together before members arrive. There are five main goals for this first group session. The first is to introduce co-facilitators and group members to one another. The second is to introduce patients to a general overview of the intervention (e.g., treatment goals, structured weekly topics, and logistics). The third is to become familiar with each patient's story of illness. The fourth is to introduce patients to an overview of this first session (e.g., Viktor Frankl's work and foundations of meaning). And the fifth goal is to share definitions of meaning and conduct the "Meaningful Moments" experiential exercise.

Introduction to Intervention

Greeting

Welcome the group and thank them for participating in this meaning-centered group psychotherapy intervention program (or research study-if you are conducting a research replication study). Example 1.1 is a sample script of what group leaders may say to welcome participants and familiarize them with the meaning-centered group intervention. Leaders are expected to have a prior understanding of this scripted format and be able to present information in their own words.

EXAMPLE 1.1

Welcome to the first meeting of our meaning-centered group psychotherapy program. It is a program that we have developed that is inspired by the work of Viktor Frankl, the author of Man's Search for Meaning *and a number of other books on the subject of finding a sense of meaning in life. We'll be meeting for eight weekly sessions in which we'll be discussing the concept of meaningfulness and how people find a sense of meaning and purpose both in general and also specifically in relation to having a diagnosis of cancer. Terms like "meaning" and "purpose" can be rather vague, which is why we will include some specific exercises as well as a lot of discussion of the concepts that come up and how they relate to people's actual experiences.*

Introductions

Co-facilitators should briefly introduce themselves (e.g., name, credentials, staff position, how long they've been working in field). They should then encourage group members to *briefly* share the following information: (1) name, (2) where they're from, (3) married/children, and (4) one or two things that are most meaningful to them. Please refer to Example 1.2 for a sample script. This should take between ten and fifteen minutes, depending on group size.

EXAMPLE 1.2

Today, we will start with an introduction to the group, getting oriented to each other and to the group's format, as well as a brief introduction to the concept of meaning. In general, we may start sessions with a brief description of the concept to be explored, to be followed by exercises and more open-ended group discussions. Sometimes there will be homework or topics to think about between sessions. One way to facilitate your understanding of our approach to meaning is by reading Frankl's Man's Search for Meaning. *Copies are available as a print book, an e-book, or as an audio version to listen to.*

Treatment Goals

The goal of these sessions is to help group members target what is meaningful in their lives, and offer ways to maintain a sense of meaning, purpose, and value in life while they're living through their individual and collective cancer experiences. These sessions are not meant to feel like traditional psychotherapy. They will be more of a mutual learning experience between all of the members, much like a "learning partnership" where members will be learning from one another. It will involve weekly experiential exercises and some homework assignments (e.g., reading) that are meant to help members learn more about the ways in which they can tap into what's meaningful in their lives.

Ground Rules

Because meaning is very individual and can even be quite intimate, ask that group members attentively listen, without passing judgment or leaping in to give advice or try to fix things. Request that each member be sensitive to others' stories and be open to what people want/need to express. Refer members to Handout 1.1, "Group Guidelines."

Logistics

Briefly discuss intervention logistics with the group. Inform them that they will be meeting for eight sessions (1.5 hours per session) and will cover a specific weekly topic (Handout 1.2, "Structured Weekly Topics"). Facilitators want the group to feel that they can depend each week on a consistent meeting time, so each session will begin promptly at _____ and end promptly at _____.

Overview of Session Topics

Handout 1.2, "Structured Weekly Topics," offers an overview and understanding of the general framework and themes of this meaning-centered intervention.

The Therapist Provides an Overview of the Trajectory of the Intervention

Session 1 will focus on the basic "concepts and sources of meaning," both in general and specifically related to cancer. Session 2 will center on "cancer and meaning," focusing on each group member's sense of identity before and after their cancer diagnosis. Sessions 3 and 4 will explore "historical sources of meaning" based on the theme "Life as a Legacy"—a legacy that's been given (via the past), a legacy that is lived (via the present), and a legacy that is given (via the future). Session 5 will address "attitudinal sources of meaning" through "encountering life's limitations" and how such limitations may affect finding meaning in the face of cancer. Session 6 will discuss "creative sources of meaning" through ways members have created and taken responsibility for their lives via the world of family, work, community, and so forth. Session 7 will explore "experiential sources of meaning" by way of "connecting with life through beauty, humor, and the lightness of being alive. Session 8, the final session, will give members a chance to reflect on their group experience and to explore hopes for the future.

Introduction to Viktor Frankl's Meaning-Centered Work

As mentioned, this meaning-centered intervention is inspired and based, in part, on an adaptation of Viktor Frankl's work, including concepts he popularized in his book *Man's Search for Meaning*. See Handout 1.3, "Individual Meaning-Centered Psychotherapy."

Basic Concepts of Meaning in Frankl's Work

Three central themes of Frankl's work are the basic concepts in individual meaning-centered psychotherapy.

1. The Will to Meaning: The need to find meaning in our existence is a basic primary motivating force shaping human behavior. Meaning-making is a defining characteristic of human beings.

2. Life Has Meaning: Frankl believed that life has meaning and never ceases to have meaning, or the potential for meaning, from the first moments of life up until the last, though what is meaningful may sometimes change over time as people's circumstances change. Perhaps more broadly, in meaning-centered psychotherapy we have adapted this concept as follows: The possibility to create or experience meaning exists throughout our lives, even in the last months, weeks, days, or even hours of life. If we feel that life is "meaningless" it is not because there is no meaning in our lives (or no possibility of creating or experiencing meaning), it is because we have become disconnected from meaning or so demoralized that we see no possibility of creating or experiencing meaning. The imperative then is to constantly "search" for meaning and meaningful moments. This search may be as important as actually arriving at a meaningful destination. Many existential philosophers felt that there is no externally given meaning to human existence and that it is left solely to human beings to create the meaning in their lives. Others, like Frankl, held out the possibility of some "ultimate" externally determined meaning given to human beings by a creator, suggesting that it is our responsibility to "search" for this ultimate meaning to our lives.

3. Freedom of Will: We have the "freedom" to find meaning in our existence and to choose our attitude toward suffering. One can think of "suffering" as the experience of encountering profound limitations and uncertainty. While there are many aspects of suffering that we have no control over, Frankl suggests that perhaps the last ultimate vestige of freedom that we have as human beings is to consider and choose our attitude toward suffering, even when almost every other freedom has been taken from us. Frankl came to this realization in concentration camp. Certainly cancer illness and treatment are not to be compared to a concentration camp experience; however, cancer illness and treatment do in fact impose significant limitations, uncertainty and suffering which requires relinquishing a great deal of control. The concept of freedom of will suggests that, despite all the limitations, uncertainty and suffering imposed by cancer, one does have the freedom to choose how one responds to these aspects of the cancer experience.

Existential Facts of Life

Three facts of life that everyone has to deal with sooner or later are guilt, suffering, and death. "Guilt" here refers to existential guilt: the fact that none of us ever truly lives our life to its unique and fullest potential. So there are unfinished life tasks, regrets, and shortcomings that produce this existential guilt. The task of dying is to relieve this guilt by completing life tasks, asking for forgiveness, forgiving oneself for being imperfectly human, trying to create a coherent sense of meaning of one's life, accepting who you are, and hopefully accepting the life one has lived. Suffering is experienced whenever we encounter any limitation or infringement on our freedom, and death is the ultimate limitation. On the one hand, all these issues can cause distress and make life seem meaningless. On the other hand, they can be sources for finding meaning in life. Frankl quotes the philosopher Nietzsche, who wrote, "He who has a why to live for can bear with almost any how." While sooner or later everyone must confront these existential issues, receiving a cancer diagnosis may bring them into much greater focus—sooner and more intensively.

Sources of Meaning: What Do We Mean by Meaning?

Introduce group members to the sources of meaning that will be explored throughout this meaning-centered intervention. There are at least four basic sources of meaning (See Handout 1.4, "Sources of Meaning").

1. Meaning occurs in a historical context. Historical sources of meaning involve our legacy (i.e., "Life as a Legacy").

2. Attitudinal sources refer to the attitude that one takes toward "encountering life's limitations" (e.g., personal adversity, physical pain, or emotional suffering). Karl Jaspers described suffering as the human experience of encountering any limitation, with death being the ultimate limitation. Frankl highlights the process of choosing our attitude toward suffering or limitations by turning what appears to be a personal human tragedy into a personal triumph.

3. Creative sources of meaning include work or artistic pursuits or causes that are derived from creating one's life and living to one's full and unique potential, through "actively engaging in life."

4. Experiential sources involve "connecting with life" through relationships (to self and loved ones), through beauty in nature or art or through humor. Connection/connectedness is essential to survival of the human specific and is the essence of the human experience. Experiential sources of meaning are those aspects of meaning that we human beings derive from experiencing the world with all of our senses, resulting in a sense of awe and meaning.

While it may sound somewhat abstract, in reality what is perceived as meaningful is very specific to each person and speaks to what each of us individually feels is important in life—our beliefs, our values, our hopes for the future. Even more, a sense of meaning cannot be expected to spontaneously arise on its own, but instead each of us is vested with the responsibility of searching for meaning and finding those responsibilities, experiences, and roles in life for which we are each irreplaceable. Each of us must confront what life is demanding of us at each moment and must choose how we respond to what life gives us, both joyful and challenging. Meaning, in fact, is created and experienced "moment to moment". What we hope to help foster in this group is the development of a sense of those values, attitudes, and experiences that imbue a sense of meaning and purpose in life. We hope members will develop skills that they'll continue to use after the group ends, to help them live a meaningful life for as long as possible.

A facilitator of meaning-centered psychotherapy must be committed to the belief that the potential for experiencing meaning always exists, no matter what the circumstances. Our role as therapists is to affirm the fact that we always have the possibility to experience meaning in life, even in the last moments of life. It is always our obligation to help the patients to be free to become their authentic selves. When a patient cannot see how she can find true meaning in life anymore, the therapist must believe in the possibility of rediscovering and reconnecting with meaning. Meaning, or the possibility of experiencing meaning, exists from the very first moment in life to the very last, and never ceases to exist.

Facilitators may now offer a brief overview of the first session, which encompasses two main goals: (1) introducing members to one another through their respective "cancer stories," and (2) introducing the basic definitions of meaning to the group. At this point, it is important to transition into each member's "cancer story" by asking members to attentively listen and become aware of how others have lived through their cancer experience and how members might personally relate to details of other's stories.

Patients' Cancer Stories

Facilitators should allow about thirty minutes (depending on group size) for members to share their personal stories of cancer, beginning with initial diagnosis and proceeding as they see fit from there.

Patients' Definitions of Meaning

Before offering the study's definitions of meaning, facilitators should encourage members to briefly express what "meaning means" to them—in their own words and on their own terms. No more than fifteen minutes should be spent on this brief exploration.

Study's Definitions of Meaning

Facilitators should smoothly transition from members' definitions of meaning to the study's definitions of meaning (refer to Handout 1.5, "Definitions of Meaning"). Designate one or two members to read the definitions out loud to the group. Then ask the group to briefly reflect on specific definition themes that stood out to them.

At this point facilitators should try to briefly relate definition themes back to patients' cancer stories and personal definitions of meaning in a purposeful way. Acknowledge how specific concepts and sources of meaning may relate back to their own experiences and illness narratives.

Experiential Exercise

The experiential exercise "Meaningful Moments" (Exercise 1.1) will help concretize the concept of meaning for participants through identifying meaningful moments in their lives. Again, members should be asked to attentively listen to other members' meaningful experiences and see how they may or may not relate to them. Allow about thirty minutes for exercise exploration.

Time permitting, group leaders should return to Handout 1.4, "Sources of Meaning," and make reference to ways in which the stories members shared reflect specific sources of meaning in their own lives. Facilitators should be aware of the meaning source categories and should be prepared to reframe specific examples given by participants into their source categories.

Examples are:

REALIZING CREATIVE VALUES: Work, projects, professional achievements, artistic endeavors (hobbies: writing, painting, sculpting), causes, good deeds, and so forth. When realizing creative values, one is *actively creating* something (e.g., work of art, career) and feeling a sense of pride or accomplishment toward this investment.

REALIZING EXPERIENTIAL VALUES: Relationships, family matters, beloved pets, being in love, appreciating the beauty of something or someone, appreciating nature or artistic endeavors. Realizing experiential values involves a more *passive appreciation* or joy in witnessing art, such as listening to a symphony or being inspired by a special book or sunset on the beach.

REALIZING HISTORICAL VALUES: Our personal story, the story of our family, things we have accomplished and learned about life that we can pass on to others—our lasting legacy.

REALIZING ATTITUDINAL VALUES: How one has coped with unavoidable suffering, that is, difficult or tragic situations, over which one both objectively and subjectively does not have control. Examples are feeling pride in getting through a painful situation (e.g., chemo treatment), a feeling of "rising above" difficult circumstances or of simply getting through a difficult day or time.

Session Wrap-Up

Remind the group of their homework assignment (see Homework 1.1 and Homework/Experiential Exercise 1.2) to start reading Viktor Frankl's *Man's Search for Meaning* (i.e., part 1) and to think about "Meaning and Cancer", by examining their identity before and after their cancer diagnosis, so that in the next session they'll be able to explore their homework in light of the theme of Session 2, "Cancer and Meaning." Suggest to the group members that they should continue to read as much of *Man's Search for Meaning* as they can over the duration of the group intervention. Ask if there are any final comments or questions before ending. The therapist should wrap up the session by reminding the group of the day/time of next session (see Handout 1.6). Thank the group members for making the commitment to attend the group sessions.

Therapist Adherence Checklist and Group Process Note

Session 1: Concepts and Sources of Meaning

☐ Introduced oneself and intervention overview

☐ Introduced concepts and sources of meaning

☐ Group members told cancer story

☐ Discussed group members' and study's definitions of meaning

☐ Patients engaged in "Meaningful Moments" exercise

☐ Provided overview of following week's session—"Cancer and Meaning"

☐ Discussed homework: read first chapter of Frankl's *Man's Search for Meaning*

Relevant themes:

Group:

Individual Members:

Group Member A:

Group Member B:

Group Member C:

Group Member D:

Group Member E:

Group Member F:

Group Member G:

Explanations for omitted session components:

Therapist Adherence to Intervention Self-Rating
(Rated 0 = "Not Adherent" to 10 = "Extremely Adherent")

Rating:
Next session scheduled for: **Date:**   **Time:**

Cancer and Meaning

Identity before and after Cancer Diagnosis

*We must never forget that we may find meaning in life even when
confronted with a hopeless situation, when facing a fate that cannot be
changed. For what then matters is to bear witness to the uniquely human
potential at its best, which is to transform a personal tragedy into a
triumph, to turn one's predicament into a human achievement. When we
are no longer able to change a situation, such as inoperable cancer, we are
challenged to change ourselves.*

Viktor Frankl, *Man's Search for Meaning* (1957, p. 116)

Session 2 Overview

1. **GROUP PERSONAL/MEDICAL CHECK-IN**

2. **PROCESSING SESSION 1**
   - Reflection on first session
   - Reflection on homework assignment re: Frankl book or video

3. **Frankl's *"Cancer and Meaning"* Figure**
   - Reference back to 1st Session re: *concepts of meaning* (e.g., ways
     to find, maintain, and enhance meaning if/when it has been lost)

4. **Explore Exercise—RE: *"Identity and Who I am"* (30 MIN)**

5. **Explore Exercise—RE: *"Identity and Cancer"* (30 MIN)**

6. **Session Wrap-Up**
   - Wrap up session by briefly reflecting on session theme, "Cancer
     and Meaning," and how it relates to patients' sense of identity
     in relation to self and others through their cancer experiences.
   - Introduce Session 3 theme ("Historical Context of Meaning"),
     and give homework assignment for following session.

Session Preparation

Co-facilitators should briefly meet ten to fifteen minutes before the session begins to prepare for the group. During this time, they should make sure they have the exercise and homework handouts available, and should ensure that the audiotape and/or video recorder are working properly (if this is being done for research or training purposes).

Session Goals

During this preparatory period, facilitators should reflect on and briefly discuss the topic and goals for this session together before members arrive. The main goal for Session 2 is to reintroduce the basic concepts and sources of meaning from the prior session, and to explore the topic of "Cancer and Meaning" in light of the guiding theme: "Identity before and after Cancer Diagnosis." By the end of Session 2, group members should have a general understanding of what one's authentic sense of identity is and the impact cancer has had on it.

Group Check-In

Welcome members back to the second session of meaning-centered group therapy. Inform them that before each session gets under way there will be a brief "check-in" to see how members are doing personally and medically since the last session. This short session check-in should last no longer than five to ten minutes; facilitators need to gently limit how much time is spent discussing medical and other issues, and when possible, should highlight connections between information shared and themes of meaning.

Process Session 1

Briefly review the major themes (and handouts) of Session 1 regarding definitions and sources of meaning. Ask members if they had given any thought to these themes over the prior week, and if so—how? This should last between five and ten minutes.

Homework Reflection

Remind members of Viktor Frankl's work (Handout 1.3) and ask them to reflect on themes that they personally related to from his book *Man's Search for Meaning*. This homework reflection should take five to ten minutes, depending on group size and interest.

Introduction to Session 2: "Cancer and Meaning"

At this point leaders should be able to transition from themes shared in homework reflection on Frankl's work to the session's theme, namely, "Cancer and Meaning: Identity before and after Cancer Diagnosis." Show members the "Cancer and Meaning" handout (Handout 2.1) and identify how cancer may affect peoples' lives.

Suffering occurs any time we, as humans, confront a limitation. Cancer presents many such obstacles/limitations, and death is the ultimate limitation. Suffering may be understood as multidimensional in nature, involving such dimensions as physical pain, mental anguish, and emotional/spiritual suffering. In times of suffering, people may become disconnected from meaning, value, and purpose in life. Frankl suggests the possibility that meaning never ceases to exist and describes the potential of humans to find meaning in suffering and in life itself. By drawing on sources of meaning as resources to reconnect with meaning (refer to Handout 1.4), participants are encouraged to be aware of the fact that, even when it appears that one has no control over cancer, one still has control over the attitude one takes toward cancer. The last vestige of human freedom is the ability to choose one's attitude in the face of suffering. By choosing one's attitude toward suffering, one can learn to not only find but also maintain and even enhance meaning and purpose in life as they face their respective cancer experiences.

Exercise: Identity and Cancer

In the previous session, members were asked to share meaningful moments that made a special impact on their lives. One's identity is composed in many ways of those things that one finds meaningful. This session will help clarify participants' authentic sense of identity, in and through meaningful experiences. This session's experiential exercises will explore what it is about such experiences that made them meaningful to that individual. What made these personal experiences meaningful gives us a glimpse into each member's personal sense of identity. In order to reflect on the origins of meaning in each member's life, it is important to start with their own understanding of who they are. Through the following exercise, encourage participants to explore and discover a little more about who they are vis-à-vis their *authentic* sense of self, and how cancer may have impacted these answers. Ask members to reflect on and share their answers to the questions asked in Homework/Experiential Exercise 1.2 regarding their sense of identity. Facilitators should leave the remaining hour to Homework/Experiential Exercise 1.2 with the group.

✓ *Therapist Note*: What will likely be most common and notable about group members' responses in these experiential exercises is that the core aspects of their identity (i.e., those elements and sources of meaning that contribute to their sense of identity) after cancer are strikingly constant and similar to their identity before cancer. Therapists should attend to these themes and highlight them as characteristics that are authentic and immutable to the patients' sense of self despite the experience of cancer.

Identity is often a function of the roles one fulfills in life (e.g., parent, spouse, etc.). These roles are often anchored in physical "actions" that define the role, typically such actions as working to financially support the family, sexual intimacy, playing football with a teenage son. Cancer illness and treatment can make these actions impossible, and so one's identity based on these roles is significantly altered. A helpful technique that we use in MCP is to help patients move from "ways of doing" to "ways of being" a parent or spouse. One is still a father if one can sit on the couch, watching the football game, sharing the experience with your son and talking about your love and pride and hopes and dreams for your son, even if one is too fatigued to throw a football around in the backyard.

In the remaining five to ten minutes of the session, bring closure to the group by briefly reflecting on the session theme, "Cancer and Meaning," and how it relates to members' sense of identity and their respective cancer experiences. Ask members if they have any final thoughts or comments they'd like to share regarding this topic before concluding the group. Briefly introduce Session 3 topic, "Historical Sources of Meaning" and the theme: "Life as a Legacy." The following session will explore the dimensions of "personal legacy," and the "legacy that has been given (past)." Provide Homework/Experiential Exercise 2.1, which is to be completed for Session 3.

Ask the group if they have any final comments or questions regarding the session or homework assignment before ending. Close the session by reminding the group of the day/time of the next session. Thank the group members for coming, and let them know that you look forward to seeing them again for Session 3.

Therapist Adherence Checklist and Group Process Note

Session 2: Identity before and after Cancer Diagnosis

☐ Conducted check-in

☐ Processed Session 1

☐ Reviewed HW (begin reading *MSFM*)

☐ Was HW (begin reading *MSFM*) completed?

☐ Referenced *concepts of meaning* introduced in Session 1

☐ Group members engaged in "Identity before Cancer" exercise

☐ Group members engaged in "Identity after Cancer" exercise

☐ Provided overview of following week's session—"Historical Sources of Meaning"

☐ Discussed homework: reflection on experiential exercises for Session 3

Relevant themes:

Group:

Individual Members:

Group Member A:

Group Member B:

Group Member C:

Group Member D:

Group Member E:

Group Member F:

Group Member G:

Explanations for omitted session components:

Therapist Adherence to Intervention Self-Rating
(Rated 0 = "Not Adherent" to 10 = "Extremely Adherent")

Rating:
Next session scheduled for: Date: Time:

Historical Sources of Meaning

"Life as a Legacy" That Has Been Given

Session 3 Overview

1. GROUP PERSONAL/MEDICAL CHECK-IN

2. INTRODUCE SESSION 3 TOPIC: "HISTORICAL SOURCES OF MEANING"
   - Briefly explore "meaning in historical context" (re: past, present, and future meanings of one's life)
   - Introduce the theme "Life as Legacy" and ask members to briefly define the concept of "legacy" on their own terms

3. EXERCISE: "LIFE AS A LEGACY" THAT HAS BEEN GIVEN
   - Past Legacy: Regarding familial lineage, upbringing, traditions, and so forth

4. SESSION WRAP-UP
   - Wrap up session by briefly reflecting on session theme.
   - Introduce Session 4 theme ("Life as a Legacy That One Lives and Will Give"), and offer homework assignment (Homework 3.1) for following session.

Session Preparation

Co-facilitators should briefly meet ten to fifteen minutes before the session begins to prepare for the group. During this time, they should make sure they have the exercise and homework handouts available, and should ensure that the audiotape and/or video recorder are working properly (if this is being done for research or training purposes).

Session Goals

During this preparatory period, facilitators should reflect on and briefly discuss the theme and goals for this session together before members arrive. The main goal for Session 3 is to introduce and explore the topic of "Historical Sources of Meaning" and the guiding theme "Life as a Legacy." Members should be given the chance to describe their personal understanding of "legacy" on their own terms, before leaders explore the concept of "legacy" in historical context (e.g., past, present, and future legacy). By the end of Session 3, group members should have a solid understanding of "the legacy that has been given" to them (via: **past** familial upbringing, family values, meaningful relationships and memories that have shaped their lives).

Group Check-In

Welcome members back to the third session of meaning-centered group therapy. Begin the session by briefly checking in to see how members are doing personally and medically since the last session. This short session check-in should last no longer than ten minutes.

Process Session 2

Briefly return to Handout 1.2 on the weekly topics and draw attention to the progression of session topics through to today's Session 3, "Historical Sources of Meaning." Ask members if they had given any thought to the prior Session 2 theme regarding "Cancer and Meaning" over the last week, and if so—how? This should last no longer than five to ten minutes.

Homework Reflection

Remind members of the homework assignment that was offered at the end of Session 2 (Homework/Experiential Exercise 2.1, "Life as a Legacy That Has Been Given"). Begin initial reflection on the general topic of "Life as a Legacy," and ask members what the term "legacy" means to them. Use this discussion as a segue for introducing today's session of "Life as a Legacy That's Been Given" (via: past experiences). The homework reflection should last between fifteen and twenty minutes, depending on group size and interest.

Introduction to Session 3: "Historical Sources of Meaning"

At this point, leaders should smoothly integrate an introduction of the session topic: "Historical Sources of Meaning" into a group exploration of the session homework/exercise.

> ✓ *Therapist Note*: Example 3.1 is a sample script of one way in which therapists might choose to proceed into a brief discussion of the "historical context of meaning." Therapists should already have a basic understanding of this topic and be prepared to offer it in their own words and on their own terms.

EXAMPLE 3.1

*One of the features that differentiate human beings from other animals is the fact that we live in a historical context—that there is a story to our family's life and our own individual lives. In one sense, we are the lead characters, with the people around us in supporting roles, and with scenery, plots, and lessons learned. In another sense, though, we may choose to cast ourselves in the supporting role, focusing on what others have given to us in terms of values, mean to us, and need from us. Frankl, quoying Nietsche, suggested: "He who has a **why** to live for can bear with almost any how"—this **why** springs out of **who you are**, what values you have and have not yet realized, what goals you may have, what is important for you. All this comes out of the story of who you are. Thinking about the story of your life helps reflect back on what you have found meaningful or joyful, what tasks you have undertaken, and what tasks may remain to be undertaken. Telling your story connects you with the people around you and keeps you connected with them whether they are physically in your presence or not. These tasks can be in any realm— they could be stories to write, children to care for, lessons to learn or teach, relationships to attend to, artistic endeavors like painting or sculpture, and so forth. One can even find meaning in the very act of bearing witness to the events of our lives. What is important about these jobs is that they're meaningful to you.*

Looking at your life from a historical perspective is not the goal in itself, but a means to an end. For one, it helps you appreciate your own past accomplishments at the same time that it helps elucidate goals by exploring for what and to whom you feel responsible. In this session, the focus is on those aspects of your legacy that were given to you, that you did not choose. For example, who your parents were and the values they imparted, the environment in which you were raised, limitations of your origin that you transcended. One's legacy given may have been positive or negative. The purpose of this session is to understand what you have been given by life, how that has influenced who you are as a person, and your life story, and how you have responded to this legacy that you have been given.

At this point, therapists should refer group members' attention to the session's experiential exercise. After giving them an opportunity to write down their responses or add additional comments to what they may have done outside of session for homework, invite open discussion for members to share their responses to Homework/Experiential Exercise 2.1 with one another. This exercise discussion should last for the remainder of the session.

✓ **Therapist Note**: Through this exercise, members should be given the opportunity to explore and express meaningful past experiences, in order to get an overall feel for the historical context of their living legacy. The "legacy that has been given" is often multidimensional in nature: for example, biological/genetic legacy, familial legacy, developmental legacy, cultural legacy, and so on. Such past legacy is immutable and cannot be undone. It is a part of who we are, whether we like it or not. For some, this exercise exploration will be a "nice trip down memory lane," while for others this might be an opportunity to share early negative experiences related to unmet needs, loss, or disappointments that may have meaningfully impacted their lives, as well. Group leaders should gently remind members to attentively listen to other's stories ("the good, the bad, and the ugly"), without passing judgment or offering quick fixes. Bearing witness to each person's early story may be experienced as quite comforting and transformative for those who yearn to be heard.

The role of facilitators should be to promote elaboration of themes of meaning that arise, to connect mutual themes of meaning expressed by group members, and to identify sources of meaning in the context of the discussion.

In the remaining five to ten minutes of the session, bring closure to the group by briefly reflecting on the session theme, "Life as a Legacy," and how it relates to members' reflections on the "legacy they have been given." Ask members if they have any final thoughts or comments they'd like to share regarding this topic before concluding the group. Briefly introduce Session 4 topic, as a continuation of "Historical Sources of Meaning" by way of the theme: "Life as a Legacy—That One Lives and Will Give." The following session will explore the dimensions of "personal legacy," with special emphasis on their present and future "living legacy." Provide the homework assignment for the next session (Homework/Experiential Exercise 3.1), which is essentially preparing members for the exact exercise they will explore in Session 4 regarding living and giving their legacy.

Session 3: Historical Sources of Meaning

☐ Conducted check-in

☐ Processed Session 2, "Cancer and Meaning"

☐ Reviewed HW on Session 3 experiential exercise

☐ Was HW reflecting on Session 3 experiential exercise completed?

☐ Briefly explored "meaning in a historical context"

☐ Briefly explored "life as a legacy that has been given"

☐ Patient engaged in "Legacy That Has Been Given" exercise

☐ Provided overview of following week's session—"Historical Sources of Meaning: Life as a Legacy That One Lives and Will Give"

☐ Discussed homework: "Share your Legacy" and preparation for Session 4 Experiential Exercise

Relevant themes:

Group:

Individual Members:

Group Member A:

Group Member B:

Group Member C:

Group Member D:

Group Member E:

Group Member F:

Group Member G:

Explanations for omitted session components:

Therapist Adherence to Intervention Self-Rating
(Rated 0 = "Not Adherent" to 10 = "Extremely Adherent")

Rating:

Next session scheduled for: **Date:**   **Time:**

Historical Sources of Meaning

"Life as a Legacy" That One Lives and Will Give

The meaning of life differs from man to man, from day to day and from hour to hour. What matters, therefore, is not the meaning of life in general but rather the specific meaning of a person's life at a given moment.

One should not search for an abstract meaning of life. Everyone has his own specific vocation or mission in life to carry out a concrete assignment, which demands fulfillment. Therein he cannot be replaced, nor can his life be repeated. Thus, everyone's task is as unique as is his specific opportunity to implement it.

Viktor Frankl, *Man's Search for Meaning* (1959, p. 113)

Session 4 Overview

1. GROUP PERSONAL/MEDICAL CHECK-IN

2. PROCESS: SESSION 3
   - Reflection: third session (re: "life as legacy that has been given")

3. INTRODUCE SESSION 4 TOPIC: "HISTORICAL SOURCES OF MEANING: LIFE AS A LEGACY THAT ONE LIVES AND WILL GIVE"
   - Briefly explore "Meaning in Historical Context" (re: past, present, and future meanings of one's life)
   - Briefly review concept of "Life as a Legacy" re: present and future legacy

4. EXPERIENTIAL EXERCISE
   - Present Legacy: Reflection on meaningful activities and accomplishments
   - Future Legacy: Reflection on life lessons and what will be passed on

> 5. SESSION WRAP-UP
> - Wrap up session by briefly reflecting on session theme.
> - Introduce Session 4 theme ("Meaning Derived from Attitudinal Values"), and offer homework assignment (e.g., share life story with loved one[s]) for following session.

Session Preparation

Co-facilitators should briefly meet ten to fifteen minutes before the session begins to prepare for the group. During this time, they should make sure they have the exercise and homework handouts available, and should ensure that the audiotape and/or video recorder are working properly (if this is being done for research or training purposes).

Session Goals

During this preparatory period, facilitators should take some time to reflect on and briefly discuss the theme and goals for this session together before members arrive. The main goal for Session 4 is to continue to explore the topic "Historical Sources of Meaning" and the guiding theme "Life as a Legacy." Leaders should pick up where they left off from Session 3 by continuing to explore the concept of "legacy" in historical context (e.g., past, present, future). By the end of Session 4, group members should have a solid understanding of "the legacy that they live and will give" via **present** roles and accomplishments, and **future** lessons and wisdom they hope to pass on.

Group Check-In

Welcome members back to the fourth session of meaning-centered group therapy. Begin the session by briefly checking in to see how members are doing personally and medically since the last session. This short session check-in should last no longer than ten minutes.

Process Session 3

Briefly return to Handout 1.2 on the weekly topics and draw attention to the progression of session topics through to today's Session 4, "Historical Sources of Meaning." Ask members if they had given any thought to the prior Session 3 theme over the last week ("Historical Sources of Meaning" in terms of "the legacy they were given"), and if so—how? This should last no longer than five to ten minutes.

Homework Reflection

Remind members of Homework/Experiential Exercise 3.1 that was offered at the end of Session 3. Continue reflection on the general topic of "Life as a Legacy" and ask members if their original ideas regarding "legacy" have shifted or changed since having the opportunity to personally explore the historical dimensions of this theme in the context of their lives. Use this discussion as a purposeful segue for introducing today's session of "Life as a Legacy That One Lives and Will Give" (via: present and future experiences).

Introduction to Session 4 "Historical Sources of Meaning"

At this point, leaders should transition from themes shared in the last session and recent homework reflection to this session's (continuation) of the topic "Historical Sources of Meaning" in light of the guiding theme: "Life as a Legacy That One Lives and Will Give." Therapists should reflect on themes presented in the prior session (refer to Session 3 sample script, if needed). The goal here is to guide members to begin to witness their living legacy as a cohesive whole, by integrating **past** memories, with **present** accomplishments, toward **future** contributions. The narrative or text of our lives must always be understood in the *context* of the whole, from the beginning to the middle and on to the end of our life story—"It will all be fine in the end. If it is not fine yet, then it is not the end."

While the legacy we have been given cannot be changed, the legacy that we *live* and *will give* are continually open to possibilities of growth and renewal. The "legacy we live" in the **present** is dynamic and ever changing. It encompasses meaningful roles, activities, and accomplishments that have made life worth living. Examples may be: the *legacy one is living* as a parent or grandparent or the *legacy one lives* in one's career or in one's community (e.g., volunteering or special deeds/causes). The point to remember is: the lives we are leading right now create the memories for our lasting legacy. So from this vantage point, we must begin to evaluate how the "legacy we live" in the present might impact "the legacy we will give" in the future. The meaningful questions then arise: What are the life-lessons we hope to pass on? How will we contribute to the greater whole? How will we be remembered? What will endure *beyond* me?

At this point, leaders should transition to the experiential exercise, which will allow members to explore and express their present and future legacy on their own terms. This exercise should last for the remainder of the session. Group leaders should be sure that members answer both parts of the experiential exercise, focusing first on the present moment and the "legacy that one lives," and then on the future "legacy that one will give."

Session Wrap-Up

In the remaining five to ten minutes of the session, bring closure to the group by briefly reflecting on the session theme, "Life as a Legacy," and how it relates to members' reflections on the "legacy they live and will give." Ask members if they have any final thoughts or comments they'd like to share regarding this topic before concluding the group. Briefly introduce Session 5 topic "Attitudinal Sources of Meaning" in terms of the guiding theme "Encountering Life's Limitations." The following session will explore Frankl's core concept of "choosing our attitude" in the face of life's limitations. Distribute Homework/Experiential Exercise 4.1, which relates to "Attitudinal Sources of Meaning", and Homework 4.2 to be completed for the next session, which encourages members to begin to share their life narrative story with family and friends, with particular emphasis on the legacy given by ancestors and historical events, the meaningful moments and events of the life they have created, and the life lessons learned that form the basis of the legacy they will leave.

Ask the group if they have any final comments or questions regarding the session or homework assignment before ending. Close the session by reminding the group of the day/time of the next session. Thank the group members for coming and let them know you look forward to seeing them again for Session 5.

Session 4: Historical Sources of Meaning: Life as a Legacy That One Lives and Will Give

☐ Conducted check-in

☐ Processed Session 3—Past Legacy

☐ Noted progression of time, and forecast transition session in three weeks

☐ Briefly explore present and future legacy

☐ Patients engaged in experiential exercise "Life as a Legacy That One Lives and Will Give"

☐ Provided overview of following week's session—"Attitudinal Sources of Meaning"

Relevant themes:

Group:

Individual Members:

Group Member A:

Group Member B:

Group Member C:

Group Member D:

Group Member E:

Group Member F:

Group Member G:

Explanations for omitted session components:

Therapist Adherence to Intervention Self-Rating
(Rated 0 = "Not Adherent" to 10 = "Extremely Adherent")

Rating:
Next session scheduled for: **Date:**   **Time:**

Attitudinal Sources of Meaning

Encountering Life's Limitations

*Any attempt to restore a man's inner strength had first to succeed in showing him some future goal. Nietzsche's words, "He who has a **why** to live for can bear with almost any **how**," could be the guiding motto for all psychotherapeutic efforts.*

What was really needed was a fundamental change in our attitude toward life. . . it did not really matter what we expected from life, but rather what life expected from us. We needed to stop asking about the meaning of life, and instead to think of ourselves as those who were being questioned by life.

Viktor Frankl, *Man's Search for Meaning* (1959, pp. 84–85)

Life gives us many things. Some appear to be wonderful, and some appear to be tragic. What is most important is to utilize our freedom to choose how we respond to what life gives us.

William Breitbart, M.D.

Session 5 Overview

1. **Group personal Check-In**

2. **Processing Session 4**
   - Reflection on fourth session
   - Reflection/Review of homework assignment

3. **Introduce Session 5 Topic: "Attitudinal Sources of Meaning"**
   - Revisit "Structured Weekly Topics" handout and define progression to topic 5 (briefly reference termination process as segue to session topic)
   - Briefly explore "attitudinal sources of meaning" (re: "Encountering Life's Limitations" when facing illness or the finiteness of life)

4. **Explore Exercises**
   - Present: How members are coping with limitations re: cancer diagnosis
   - Future: How members want/hope to be remembered

5. **Session Wrap-Up**
   - Wrap up session by briefly reflecting on session theme.
   - Introduce Session 6 theme ("Creative Sources of Meaning").
   - Give homework assignment for following session and explore "legacy project."

Session Preparation

Co-facilitators should briefly meet ten to fifteen minutes before the session begins to prepare for the group. During this time, they should make sure they have the exercise and homework handouts available, and should ensure that the audiotape and/or video recorder are working properly (if this is being done for research or training purposes).

Session Goals

During this preparatory period, facilitators should reflect on and briefly discuss the theme and goals for this session together before members arrive. The main goal for Session 5 is to explore the topic "Attitudinal Sources of Meaning" and the guiding theme "Encountering Life's Limitations." Leaders should pick up where they left off from Session 4 by continuing to explore the concept of "legacy" in historical context (e.g., past, present, and future dimensions) in light of confronting the ultimate limitation of death and the lasting legacy they will leave. By the end of Session 5, group members should have a solid understanding of "attitudinal sources of meaning" based on Frankl's core theme that *our last vestige of human freedom is to choose our attitude toward suffering and life's limitations.* In simpler terms, life presents us with many circumstances that may be opportunities or limitations. While we often don't have control over what life gives us (i.e., love, cancer), we always have the freedom to choose how we respond to and the attitude we take toward what life gives us, good or bad.

Check-In

Welcome members back to the fifth session of meaning-centered group therapy. Begin the session by briefly checking in to see how members are doing personally and medically since the last session. This short session check-in should last no longer than ten minutes.

Process Session 4

Briefly return to Handout 1.2 on the weekly topics and draw attention to the progression of session topics through to today's Session 5, "Attitudinal Sources of Meaning." Ask members if they had given any thought to the prior Session 4 theme, "Present and Future Legacy," over the last week, and if so—how? This should last between five and ten minutes.

Homework Reflection

Remind members of the Homework/Experiential Exercise 4.1; and Homework 4.2 that was offered at the end of the last Session, regarding sharing their stories with loved ones. Ask them how it was to share their life history with their loved one(s). How did it feel to be attended to (i.e., heard, witnessed, or validated) while telling their stories out loud? Allow about twenty to thirty minutes for members to process their feelings regarding this homework assignment depending on how many completed homework assignment and interest level.

Introduction to Session 5: "Attitudinal Sources of Meaning"

At this point, leaders should use this session's theme, "Encountering Life's Limitations," as a quick transition point to reference the group's final session in three weeks. Ask members to briefly share any thoughts/feelings they have about the group sessions coming to an end. Again, this early discussion of the limitations of the group timeline can be a nice reflective segue toward introducing the topic of the attitude one takes toward life's limitations, "Attitudinal Sources of Meaning," and the guiding theme of "Encountering Life's Limitations."

This session will explore what it means to not only face but also transcend life's limitations. It will highlight Viktor Frankl's core theoretical belief that by *choosing our attitude* toward "suffering" and circumstances that are beyond our control (e.g., cancer and death), we may find meaning in life and find a way to "transcend" such limitations. Frankl used the term "suffering" when he described the possibility of "finding meaning through one's attitude towards suffering." "Suffering" is a complex term with many definitions. Karl Jaspers defined suffering as the human experience of encountering any limitation. In life we encounter many limitations from the mundane to the profound, for example, a dream not coming true, physical limitations, and ultimately death. Eric Cassel defined suffering as a loss of "personhood." This is best understood as the loss of one's human essence or more simply the loss of significant elements of one's identity (an identity formed by the roles one plays in life that gives life meaning). So when Frankl speaks of suffering, he is in fact speaking of the limitations imposed by events in life and the impact of these limitations on one's identity and sense of humanity. Frankl suggested that our last vestige of human freedom was the freedom to choose the attitude we take toward suffering. When all else has been stripped away (e.g., physical, mental, spiritual well-being), we still have the capacity to choose how we respond to any given circumstance.

The term "transcend" is also quite complex and often difficult to understand. In simple terms, it means to overcome or rise above limitations or obstacles in life. In fact, to transcend also involves the concept of connectedness beyond oneself, to rise above one's own individual concerns and connect to something greater than oneself. This can involve connectedness to loved ones or to values or causes or life itself, that is, those things you care most about in the world. Breitbart describes transcendence as one of three types of escalators at the airport. The ascending escalators take you up. The descending escalators take you down. But where are the transcending escalators? These are the moving walkways that connect you from one gate to another and allow you to connect with every part of the world.

> ✓ *Therapist Note*: This topic (e.g., attitude and self-transcendence) might be a difficult concept for members to grasp. Find an opportune time to offer examples or to read a brief passage from Frankl's work (See: Session 5 title page) to drive home points.

> ✓ *Therapist Note*: Example 5.1 is a sample script that introduces the existential issues related to encountering life's limitations, particularly confronting one's fate and the finiteness of life. Leaders should find their own way to explore this theme on their own terms.

EXAMPLE 5.1

Our knowledge of the finiteness of life is in part responsible for the need people have for a sense of meaning or purpose. Learning to cope with limitations is what allows us to appreciate those things that we do have. As Frankl states in Man's Search for Meaning, *". . . often, it is just such an exceptionally difficult external situation which gives man the opportunity to grow spiritually beyond himself." He viewed his own experiences during the holocaust as tests of his inner strength, and he viewed his coping with such extreme situations with a feeling of pride and accomplishment.*

The fact that we have only a limited amount of time also challenges us to make the most of the time we have. Frankl uses the metaphor of a sculptor hammering away at an as yet unshaped stone. Knowing that he has a limited amount of time to finish his work, while not knowing when exactly the deadline will be, forces him to use his time as best he can and make the most of every moment. For Frankl, the stone at which we hammer is our lives and what we hammer out is our values—creative, experiential (love, family, beauty, art) and attitudinal (how we cope with our unchangeable fates). Thus, he points out that as we cannot judge a biography by the number of pages in it but by the richness of its contents, similarly we cannot judge our lives simply by their length but by the richness of their contents. Those contents include how we live and also how we die—how we view life and death, how we cope with impending limits such as death, and the meaning we find in it.

This would be a good time to turn to the session's experiential exercise regarding "Encountering Life's Limitations" (Homework/Experiential Exercise 4.1). For the time remaining in the session, members should be given the opportunity to explore and express their thoughts/feelings regarding this sensitive subject. The exercise begins with how members are coping with their current physical and medical limitations regarding their cancer diagnosis and treatment, and then transitions into how they may face the finiteness of their lives and how they hope to be remembered.

✓ *Therapist Note*: Again, it is important to recognize the intimate nature of this topic, especially concerning death and dying. Every effort must be made to create a safe environment to explore this sensitive discussion. Members should be reminded to attentively listen without passing judgment or attempting to remedy the situation.

Session Wrap-Up

In the remaining five to ten minutes of the session, bring closure to the group by briefly reflecting on the session topic, "Attitudinal Sources of Meaning," in terms of the guiding theme "Encountering Life's Limitations." Ask members if they have any final thoughts or comments they'd like to share regarding this topic before concluding the group. Briefly introduce the Session 6 topic, "Creative Sources of Meaning" by way of "Creativity, Courage, and Responsibility." Distribute Homework/Experiential Exercise 5.1, and Homework 5.2, which nicely integrates legacy themes with the Session 6 theme, "Creativity, Courage, and Responsibility" and a reminder to create a "Legacy Project."

Ask the group if they have any final comments or questions regarding the session or homework assignment before ending. Close the session by reminding the group of the day/time of the next session. Thank the group members for coming and let them know you look forward to seeing them again for Session 6.

Session 5: Attitudinal Sources of Meaning: Encountering Life's Limitations

- ☐ Conducted check-in
- ☐ Processed Session 4—Present/Future Legacy
- ☐ Noted progression of time, and forecast transition session in three weeks
- ☐ Reviewed HW (sharing cancer story).
- ☐ Was HW (sharing cancer story) completed?
- ☐ Briefly explore "attitudinal sources of meaning" (re: finding meaning when encountering life's limitations such as facing illness or the finiteness of life)
- ☐ Patients engaged in Attitudinal Exercises 1 and 2 (how pt is coping w/ limitations re: cancer dx)
- ☐ Patients engaged in Attitudinal Exercise 3 (how does pt hope to be remembered?)
- ☐ Provided overview of following week's session—"Creative Sources of Meaning"
- ☐ Discussed homework: "Introduction to Legacy Project"

Relevant themes:

Group:

Individual Members:

Group Member A:

Group Member B:

Group Member C:

Group Member D:

Group Member E:

Group Member F:

Group Member G:

Explanations for omitted session components:

Therapist Adherence to Intervention Self-Rating
(Rated 0 = "Not Adherent" to 10 = "Extremely Adherent")

Rating:

Next session scheduled for: Date: Time:

Creative Sources of Meaning

Creativity, Courage, and Responsibility

The noblest appreciation of meaning is reserved to those people who, deprived of the opportunity to find meaning in a deed, in a work, or in love, by the very attitude which they choose to this predicament, rise above it and grow beyond themselves. What matters is the stand they take—a stand which allows for transmuting their predicament into achievement, triumph and heroism.

Viktor Frankl, *The Will to Meaning* (1969, p. 70)

As each situation in life represents a challenge to man and presents a problem for him to solve, the question of the meaning of life may actually be reversed. Ultimately, man should not ask what the meaning of his life is, but rather he must recognize that it is he who is being asked. In a word, each man is questioned by life; and he can only answer to life by answering for his own life; to life he can only respond by being responsible.

Viktor Frankl, *Man's Search for Meaning* (1959, p. 113)

Session 6 Overview

1. GROUP CHECK-IN

- Personal/Medical Check-in

2. PROCESS SESSION 5

- Reflection on fifth session
- Reflection/Review of homework assignment and check-in on legacy project

3. INTRODUCE SESSION 6 TOPIC: "CREATIVE SOURCES OF MEANING"

- Revisit Handout 1.2 on the structured weekly topics: define progression to topic 6, and reflect on termination process.
- Briefly explore "meaning derived from creativity and responsibility"

---

4. **EXPLORE EXERCISE 1: "THE ESSENCE OF CREATIVITY"**
   - Past: Creative endeavors
   - Present: Expressing self through creative process (via: courage and commitment)

5. **EXPLORE EXERCISE: "THE ESSENCE OF RESPONSIBILITY"**
   - Responsibility ~ *one's ability to respond to life*
   - Past-Present-Future Responsibilities
   - Unfinished business

6. **SESSION WRAP-UP**
   - Wrap up session by briefly reflecting on session theme.
   - Introduce Session 7 theme ("Experiential Sources of Meaning").
   - Give homework assignment for following session

Session Preparation

Co-facilitators should briefly meet ten to fifteen minutes before the session begins to prepare for the group. During this time, they should make sure they have the exercise and homework handouts available, and should ensure that the audiotape and/or video recorder are working properly (if this is being done for research or training purposes).

Session Goals

During this preparatory period, facilitators should reflect on and briefly discuss the theme and goals for this session together before members arrive. The main goal for session 6 is to introduce and explore the topic "Creative Sources of Meaning" and the guiding theme "Creativity, Courage, and Responsibility." By the end of Session 6, group members should have a solid understanding of the significance of the creative sources of meaning (creativity, courage, and responsibility) as important resources for meaning in their lives.

Group Check-In

Welcome members back to the sixth session of meaning-centered group therapy. Begin the session by briefly checking in to see how members are doing personally and medically since the last session. This short session check-in should last no longer than ten minutes.

Process Session 5

Briefly, return to Handout 1.2 on the weekly topics and draw attention to the progression of session topics through to today's Session 6, "Creative Sources of Meaning." Ask members if they had given any further thought to the Session 5 topic, "Attitudinal Sources of Meaning," over the last week, and if so—how? This might be a good time to remind them that the final session of meaning-centered psychotherapy is soon approaching. Ask members to share any thoughts/feelings surrounding the culmination of their group meetings. This discussion should last between five and fifteen minutes, depending on group size and interest.

Homework Reflection

Remind members of Homework 5.1, which was offered at the end of Session 5 with regard to creating a personal "Legacy Project." Inquire into whether people have started brainstorming about any "legacy project" ideas and whether members have any questions that will help them initiate this creative endeavor. Use this discussion as a segue for introducing today's theme, "Creativity, Courage, and Responsibility" (via: past and present experiences). Begin initial reflection on the general theme of "Creativity, Courage, and Responsibility," by asking members what these terms mean to them.

Introduction to Session 6: "Creative Sources of Meaning"

At this point, leaders should smoothly transition from themes shared in the homework reflection (e.g., creative ideas re: "legacy project") to the Session 6 topic, "Creative Sources of Meaning," and the guiding theme,

"Creativity, Courage, and Responsibility." Creativity and responsibility are core themes in Frankl's *logotherapy*, as well as in any existential discussion of human existence. Through creative endeavors we are afforded the capacity to transcend our given bounds by actively infusing something of ourselves into the world—thereby contributing to the greater whole. Creativity, through the act of creating our lives, forms our destiny. Courage is essential to the task of continuing to create a life and to fulfill one's responsibility to life in the face of the limitations of a life-threatening cancer illness. It takes courage to continue to live and have hopes and wishes and dreams when life can end. It takes courage to continue to love when all that you love can be lost. So when we speak of creative sources of meaning, we are referring to the meaning derived from creating one's life, an endeavor characterized by responsibility and requiring courage.

> ✓ *Therapist Note*: The following is a brief overview of creativity, courage, and responsibility, which is meant to help guide and inform your group discussion. We encourage leaders to use these key ideas as helpful markers, but also to bring their own creative voices to the fore when exploring such themes with their group members.

Creativity, Courage, and Responsibility: Overview

Our existence calls us to create a life, a unique life, in which we strive fulfill our full potential. We are called on to create a life of meaning, identity, direction, transformation, connection, and fulfillment, becoming a valued member of a culture or society. *Our ability to respond* to this creative calling forms the basis for taking *responsibility* (response-ability) for the life that dwells within. Creativity and responsibility, therefore, are inextricably linked. By actively responding to the call to create, we become authentically responsible for our lives. Frankl suggested, "*man should not ask what he may expect from life, but should rather understand that life expects something from him*. . . He should realize that he himself is being questioned. Life is putting this problem to him, and it is up to him to respond to these questions by being responsible; he can only answer to life by answering *for his* life" (*The Doctor and The Soul*, p. xxi). Authenticity is a relatively complex concept. In its simplest form, to be authentic is to create a life that is uniquely your own and to continue to live and grow in that life in ways that are consistent with your own unique values. Thus, authenticity is being true to the real you. The task of creating a unique life of meaning and fulfilling our responsibility to live to our full potential in a thoroughly authentic fashion is in fact often not achieved. As human beings we are imperfect and we often fail to live to our complete and fullest unique potential. We do not respond to the call of creativity every moment of our lives and so, inevitably, we fall short. We experience this as imperfection, vulnerability, flaws. We experience existential guilt when we ignore the creative calling of responsibility, or fail to respond to and take care of that life within. An example of existential guilt is embodied in the last words of Albert Einstein on his deathbed: "If only I knew more mathematics." But additionally, existential guilt is experienced when we fail to take care of the life we are responsible to care for. Guilt can be experienced as a variety of emotions, including anger, anxiety, depression, demoralization, hopelessness, and shame or can be the wellspring of empathy and the ability to love. The choice we make in our attitude toward our vulnerabilities and imperfections can lead to these very different emotional outcomes.

The beauty of creativity is that it continually gives us second chances to start over, make amends, forge new paths, traverse uncharted territories, and transcend our given bounds. The challenge of creativity is that it takes a good deal of courage, tenacity, and inner fortitude to continually risk putting oneself out there in the face of uncertainty and doubt. Rollo May, in his book *The Courage to Create* (1994), suggests that "courage is not the absence of doubt; it is the ability to move ahead in spite of it." It takes a great deal of courage to confront an advanced stage cancer diagnosis and find the energy and inner resolve *to move ahead in spite* of an uncertain future. Paul Tillich, in his book *The Courage to Be*, stresses that courage is not something that is to be sought and earned from outside oneself, it is rather something that is inherently a part of our very nature: "courage. . . is rooted in the whole breadth of human existence and ultimately in the structure of being itself" (1952, p. 1).

When we speak about patients' creative endeavors and the responsibilities they have in their lives, this is no small matter. They link their sense of meaning, identity, and worth to the activities and responsibilities that make up their lives. Here is where "the doing" of creativity intersects with the meaning of "being" alive. It is what gives them a reason to get up in the morning—a reason to move ahead into the world despite the uncertainty of their disease and fate.

Session 6—Experiential Exercise

Now that we hopefully have a basic understanding of "creativity, courage, and responsibility," it is now time to shift toward the group's understanding of these themes. Offer members the experiential exercise (Homework/Experiential Exercise 5.2), and spend the remainder of the session exploring this topic of "creative sources of meaning" on their own terms.

Session Wrap-Up

In the remaining five to ten minutes of the session, bring closure to the group by briefly reflecting on the session topic, "Creative Sources of Meaning," in terms of the guiding theme, "Creativity, Courage, and Responsibility." Ask members if they have any final thoughts or comments they'd like to share regarding this topic before concluding the group. Briefly introduce Session 7 topic, "Experiential Sources of Meaning" by way of "Connecting with Life." Distribute Homework 6.1 for the next session, which nicely integrates Session 6 themes.

Ask the group if they have any final comments or questions regarding the session or homework assignment before ending. Close the session by reminding the group of the day/time of the next session. Ask members to reflect on any thoughts or feelings that may arise over the next week regarding termination and ending the group, which they will have the opportunity to discuss and explore in the next session. Thank the group members for coming and let them know you look forward to seeing them again for Session 7.

Session 6: Creative Sources of Meaning: Creativity, Courage, and Responsibility

☐ Conducted check-in

☐ Processed Session 4—"Attitudinal Sources of Meaning"

☐ Noted progression of time, and forecast transition session in two weeks

☐ Reflections on HW (legacy project) discussed

☐ Introduced Session 6 topic—"Creative Sources of Meaning"

☐ Briefly explored "meaning derived from creativity and responsibility"

☐ Patient engaged in Experiential Exercise 1 (creative endeavors and creativity through courage and commitment)

☐ Patient engaged in Experiential Exercise 2 (responsibility, past/present/future responsibility, unfinished business)

☐ Provided overview of following week's session—"Experiential Sources of Meaning"

☐ Discussed homework: "Connecting with Life through Love, Beauty, and Humor"

Relevant themes:

Group:

Individual Members:

Group Member A:

Group Member B:

Group Member C:

Group Member D:

Group Member E:

Group Member F:

Group Member G:

Explanations for omitted session components:

Therapist Adherence to Intervention Self-Rating
(Rated 0 = "Not Adherent" to 10 = "Extremely Adherent")

Rating:
Next session scheduled for: Date: Time:

Experiential Sources of Meaning

Connecting with Life through Love, Beauty, and Humor

Love

A thought transfixed me: for the first time in my life I saw the truth as it is set into song by so many poets, proclaimed as the final wisdom by so many thinkers. The truth—that love is the ultimate and the highest goal to which man can aspire. Then I grasped the meaning of the greatest secret that human poetry and human thought and belief have to impart: the salvation of man is through love and in love.

Beauty

As the inner life of the prisoner tended to become more intense, he also experienced beauty of art and nature as never before. Under their influence he sometimes even forgot his own frightful circumstances. . . Despite that factor—or maybe because of it—we were carried away by nature's beauty, which we had missed for so long.

Humor

Humor was another of the soul's weapons in the fight for self-preservation. It is well-known that humor more than anything else in the human make-up, can afford an aloofness and an ability to rise above any situation. . . The attempt to develop a sense of humor and to see things in a humorous light is some kind of a trick learned while mastering the art of living.

Viktor Frankl, *Man's Search for Meaning* (1959, pp. 48–55)

Session 7 Overview

1. GROUP CHECK-IN
   - Personal/Medical Check-in
   - Legacy Project Check-in

2. PROCESS SESSION 6
   - Reflection on sixth session
   - Reflection/Review of homework assignment

3. INTRODUCE SESSION 7 TOPIC: "EXPERIENTIAL SOURCES OF MEANING"
   - Revisit Handout 1.2 on the structured weekly topics and define progression to topic 7 and movement toward the final, eighth session
   - Explore thoughts and feelings re: the time-limited nature of the intervention
   - Briefly explore "experiential sources of meaning" (re: "Connecting with Life through Love, Beauty, and Humor")

4. EXPLORE EXERCISE: LOVE, BEAUTY, AND HUMOR

5. SESSION WRAP-UP
   - Wrap up session by briefly reflecting on session theme.
   - Introduce Session 8 theme ("Transitions")
   - Briefly follow up re: "legacy project" progression
   - Explore thoughts/feelings re: final session

Session Preparation

Co-facilitators should briefly meet ten to fifteen minutes before the session begins to prepare for the group. During this time, they should make sure they have the exercise and homework handouts available, and should ensure that the audiotape and/or video recorder are working properly (if this is being done for research or training purposes).

Session Goals

During this preparatory period, facilitators should reflect on and briefly discuss the theme and goals for this session together before members arrive. The main goal for session 7 is to introduce and explore the topic "Experiential Sources of Meaning" by way of the guiding theme "Connecting with Life." By the end of Session 7, group members should have a solid understanding of the significance of *connecting with life through experiential sources of meaning*— particularly through the experiential sources of **love**, **beauty**, and **humor**.

Group Check-In

Welcome members back to the seventh session of meaning-centered group therapy. Begin the session by briefly checking in to see how members are doing personally and medically since the last session. This short session check-in should last no longer than ten minutes.

Process Session 6 and Termination

Briefly return to Handout 1.2 on the weekly topics and draw attention to the progression of session topics through to today's Session 7, "Experiential Sources of Meaning." Ask members if they had given any further thought to the prior Session 6 theme, "Creative Sources of Meaning," over the last week, and if so—how? This would be a good time to remind them that the next session will be their final one. Ask members to share any thoughts/feelings surrounding the ending of their group meetings. This discussion should last between five and ten minutes, depending on group size.

Homework Reflection

Remind members of the homework assignment that was offered at the end of Session 6 related to today's session regarding "connecting with life" through love, beauty, and humor. Use this initial discussion as a segue for introducing today's session theme, "Experiential Sources of Meaning." Begin initial topic reflections by briefly exploring what the experiential sources of love, beauty, and humor mean to the group.

At this point, leaders should smoothly transition from themes shared in the homework reflection to Session 7's topic, "Experiential Sources of Meaning" vis-à-vis the guiding theme "Connecting with Life" through love, beauty, and humor. Experiential sources of meaning are essentially sources of meaning that are derived from our "experience" of life. We experience life primarily through our various perceptual senses and through our emotions and thoughts. The French word for meaning is "sense." Therefore, literally, the experiential source of meaning is derived through our various perceptual sensations and our sensory system. We experience life and the meaning of life through sight, sound, taste, smell, and touch and the various aspects of the emotion of love. We experience the awesomeness of the beauty, joys, and pleasures of life through our five senses. These experiences make us feel that living and life are full of meaning. *Love* is perhaps the most profound and common source of experiential meaning. Our experience of love connects us to each other and allows us to transcend our own individual concerns. Emmanuel Levinas defined philosophy not as the love of wisdom, but the "wisdom of love" (Beals, 2007). Love can take a variety of forms; romantic, parental, filial, love of our fellow man, and love of ourselves. Love and connectedness ameliorates the existential isolation that can occur when we become disconnected from the meaning in our life. *Beauty* and *humor* connect us to the awe and joy of the experience of being alive and remind us of the meaningfulness of life. *Love* and *beauty* connect us to eternal constructs that live beyond our lifetimes.

Whereas creative and attitudinal sources of meaning require more of an *active involvement in life*, experiential sources embody more of a *passive engagement with life*. While the former sources of meaning entail more of a *dynamic "doing"* mode of *investing in life*, the latter reveals the *receptive "being"* mode of *connecting with life*. Where creative and attitudinal sources ask us to *give to life*, experiential sources call us to *give ourselves over* to the lightness of being alive—through love, art, and beauty.

✓ *Therapist Note*: Example 7.1 is a basic overview of key topic themes. We encourage leaders to familiarize themselves with these basic tenets and then give themselves over to the discussion of "connecting with life" in a meaningful manner—allowing experiential themes to emerge in organic dialogue with group members.

EXAMPLE 7.1

Experiential sources of meaning—love, beauty (i.e., art, nature), humor— allow us to transcend ourselves by being transported in contemplation within these experiences. They help us to feel a part of something greater than our- selves, like individual waves that come together to make up the ocean. Frankl describes how even in the concentration camp, he and his fellow prisoners experienced the beauty of the mountains of Salzburg or a particularly vivid sunset more richly than before because of their circumstances. They found solace in the fact that whatever their individual fates, the beauty of nature, of which they were a part, would continue beyond them.

Experiential sources of meaning are perceived in more of a passive manner of reverence and contemplation, as compared to the other two more active sources of meaning (e.g., creativity and attitude). As one surrenders to love, laughter, and the beauty of art or nature, one may lose oneself in the mo- ment of contemplation only to find oneself more authentically present to life itself. Frankl offers an example: "Imagine a music-lover sitting in the concert hall while. . . his favorite symphony resounds in his ears. He feels that shiver of emotion, which we experience in the presence of purest beauty. Suppose now that at such a moment we should ask this person whether his life has meaning. He would have to reply that it had been worthwhile living if only to experience this ecstatic moment" (The Doctor and The Soul, p. 43).

Similarly, one can feel transported by feelings of love even when the loved one is not physically present. Frankl spoke on many occasions about the enduring love he held for his wife, and how her very memory allowed him to transcend his suffering, if even for a few short moments. Humor also helps us rise above difficult circumstances by lightening the moment and allowing for healthy emotional distance from a distressing situation. Frankl went so far as to refer to humor as "another of the soul's weapons in the fight for self-preservation" (MSFM, pp. 54–55).

Session 7—Experiential Exercise

Now that we have a basic understanding of the experiential sources of meaning (and their receptive and contemplative qualities), it is now time to shift toward the group's understanding of these themes. Offer members the experiential exercise in which they discuss their answers to Homework/Experiential Exercise 6.1, and spend the remainder of the session exploring this topic of "connecting with life" through love, beauty, and humor on their own terms. Leaders should make sure that enough time is allotted to this exercise, as its very exploration may enhance a sense of renewed meaning and comfort for group members.

Session Wrap-Up

In the remaining five to ten minutes of the session, bring closure to the group by briefly reflecting on the session topic, "Experiential Sources of Meaning," in terms of the guiding theme, "Connecting with Life." Ask members if they have any final thoughts or comments they'd like to share regarding this topic before concluding the group. Remind the group that the next session will be the final group meeting. Offer members Homework/Experiential Exercise 7.1 and ask them to reflect on any thoughts or feelings that may arise over the next week regarding the ending of the group, which they will have ample opportunity to discuss and explore in the next session. Thank the group members for coming, and let them know you look forward to seeing them again for their final Session 8.

Session 7: Experiential Sources of Meaning: Connecting with Life

☐ Conducted check-in

☐ Processed Session 6—"Creative Sources of Meaning"

☐ Noted progression of time, and forecast transition session in one week

☐ Reflections on HW (connecting with love, beauty, and humor) discussed

☐ Introduced Session 7 topic—"Experiential Sources of Meaning"

☐ Briefly explored "Experiential Sources of Meaning"

☐ Patient engaged in Session 7 HW/Experiential Exercise (connecting with love, beauty, humor)

☐ Provided overview of following week's session—"Transitions: Final Reflections and Hopes for the Future"

☐ Reminded group members about "Legacy Project"

Relevant themes:

Group:

Individual Members:

Group Member A:

Group Member B:

Group Member C:

Group Member D:

Group Member E:

Group Member F:

Group Member G:

Explanations for omitted session components:

Therapist Adherence to Intervention Self-Rating
(Rated 0 = "Not Adherent" to 10 = "Extremely Adherent")

Rating:
Next session scheduled for: Date: Time:

Transitions

Final Group Reflections and Hopes for the Future

It is a peculiarity of man that he can only live by looking to the future. And this is his salvation in the most difficult moments of his existence.

Whoever was still alive had reason for hope. Whatever we had gone through could still be an asset to us in the future. And I quoted from Nietzsche: "That which does not kill me, makes me stronger."
　　　　　　Viktor Frankl, *Man's Search for Meaning* (1959, pp. 81, 89)

Session 8 Overview

1. SESSION CHECK-IN
   - Personal/Medical Check-in

2. TRANSITIONS: REFLECTION ON PREVIOUS SESSIONS

3. EXPLORATION OF LEGACY PROJECTS

4. PATIENTS' GROUP EXPERIENCE: REFLECTION AND FEEDBACK
   - What has it been like for you to go through this learning experience over these last eight sessions? Have there been any changes in the way you view your life and cancer experience having been through this process?
   - Do you feel like you have a better understanding of the sources of meaning in life and are you able to use them in your daily life? If so, how?
   - What are your hopes for the future?

5. GROUP CLOSURE
   - Wrap up intervention by briefly reflecting on meaningful moments
   - Share: thank yous and good byes
   - Reinforce: "it's been a learning experience for all of us"

Session Goals

The goals of this final session are at once simple but also complex. Leaders should help members to reflect on their group experience in light of the last seven sessions. They should facilitate dialogue and reflection around members' thoughts and feelings surrounding the finality of their group experience, in light of facing important transitions and facing their own mortality due to their cancer illness. Explore what it has been like for members to share their cancer experiences and life stories with others in the group, and to witness others' stories in return. Time should be given to share and explore members' final "Legacy Projects," as well as meaningful experiences within the group process. Time should also be allotted for patients to offer feedback regarding their group experience and hopes for the future (refer to the "Intervention Feedback" questions in Homework/Experiential Exercise 7.1).

Group Check-In

Welcome members back to their eighth and final session of meaning-centered group psychotherapy. Begin the session by briefly checking in to see how members are doing personally and medically since the last session. This should last between five and ten minutes, but may last longer if members want to share final statements with regard to their overall well-being.

Process Transition

Briefly return to Handout 1.2 on the weekly topics and draw attention to the progression of session topics through to today's eighth and final session, identifying and emphasizing weekly themes in the process. Inquire into whether members had given any thought to what this final session would be like for them over the last week. Ask members to share any thoughts/feelings they might have surrounding the finality of their group meetings. This transition discussion should last about fifteen minutes, depending on group size.

Leaders should then transition from discussing endings to exploring "new beginnings" in and through members' respective "Legacy Projects." Some may have chosen not to partake in this endeavor. Some members will state that "my life is my legacy," which is perfectly acceptable and can be reinforced as valid by the facilitators. Others may have logistic reasons for not completing the project, such as fatigue, or illness. Some may plan to create the legacy project after the group has ended, while others may have no intention to complete the project at all. Facilitators should support the members' choices to complete or not complete this project. It is their choice, after all.

> ✓ *Therapist Note*: As emphasized throughout the course of this intervention, it is important to encourage members to offer "witnessed significance" (via: attentive listening and validation) to those who are sharing their respective "Legacy Projects." This final feeling of having their legacy meaningfully witnessed and validated by their fellow group members may be a comforting and transformative experience that members may carry with them beyond the group.

Intervention Feedback

Leaders should use the remaining time in this final session to encourage members' feedback regarding the overall intervention, as well as to reflect on their hopes for the future. Refer to Homework/ Experiential Exercise 7.1, which includes questions to prompt intervention feedback and dialogue.

Session Wrap-Up

In the remaining five to ten minutes of the session, bring closure to the group by briefly reflecting on meaningful experiences, moments, or memories from their group experience. Ask members if they have any final thoughts or comments they'd like to share before bringing final closure to the group. Thank each member for being a meaningful part of this group experience and for the moments shared and the "mutual learning experiences" that were offered by all along the way.

Finally, expressions of gratitude and a reflection by the facilitators on the legacy created within the group are shared. Often it is useful for facilitators to remark on moments of courage, moments of connectedness, and moments of self-care. It is not uncommon for facilitators to acknowledge the ways in which they have been impacted by group members, the honor and privilege of sharing in these intimate moments at a critical stage in patients' lives, and affirm that the group members will not be forgotten.

A Final Meaning-Centered Statement

A reader can only apply what he has found convincing.
You cannot persuade others of anything
of which you are not convinced yourselves!
This particularly applies to the [therapist's] conviction
That life does have meaning
And that it is even unconditionally meaningful,
Up to its last moment,
To one's last breath,
And that death itself may be endowed with meaning.

We may redefine the helping professions
as called upon more specifically to help their patients
in the basic and ultimate human aspiration
of finding a meaning in their lives.
And by so doing, those who belong to the helping professions
retroactively find a vocation and mission themselves,
for their own lives:
I have seen the meaning of my life
in helping others to see in their lives a meaning.

Viktor Frankl, *The Will to Meaning* (1969, p. 160)

Therapist Adherence Checklist and Group Process Note

Session 8: Transitions: Reflection and Hopes for Future

☐ Conducted check-in

☐ Processed Session 7—"Experiential Sources of Meaning"

☐ Discussed "Legacy Project"

☐ Patient engaged in Session 8 Experiential Exercise (reflections and feedback)

☐ Wrap-up and Closure: therapist shared *thank yous and good byes*

Relevant themes:

Group:

Individual Members:

Group Member A:

Group Member B:

Group Member C:

Group Member D:

Group Member E:

Group Member F:

Group Member G:

Explanations for omitted session components:

Therapist Adherence to Intervention Self-Rating
(Rated 0 = "Not Adherent" to 10 = "Extremely Adherent")

Rating:
Next session scheduled for: Date: Time:

References

Albom, M. (1997). *Tuesdays with Morrie.* Random House, New York.

Beals, C. (2007). *Levinas and the Wisdom of Love.* Baylor University Press, Waco, TX.

Frankl, V.F. (1955/1986). *The Doctor and the Soul.* Random House, New York.

Frankl, V.F. (1959/1992). *Man's Search for Meaning* (4th ed.). Beacon Press, Boston.

Frankl, V.F. (1969/1988) *The Will to Meaning: Foundations and Applications of Logotherapy,* Expanded Edition. Penguin Books, New York.

Frankl, V. F. (1975/1997). *Man's Search for Ultimate Meaning.* Plenum Press, New York.

Frankl, V.F. (1988). *The Will to Meaning: Foundations and Applications of Logotherapy.* New American Library, New York.

Jaspers, K. (1955). *Reason and Existenz.* Translated by William Earle. Noonday Press, New York.

May, R. (1994). *The Courage to Create.* Norton, New York.

Tillich, P. (1952). *The Courage to Be.* Yale University Press, New Haven, CT.

Yalom, I.D. (1980). *Existential Psychotherapy.* Basic Books, New York.

Handout 1.1

Group Guidelines

1. *Confidentiality/Privacy*:
   - It is important to us that you feel a sense of comfort and security in freely sharing your stories and experiences in this group. We ask that members respect others' privacy by not sharing these stories outside the confines of the group environment.
   - Each session will be audio- and/or videotaped, for quality assurance purposes. All recorded information will be kept in a secure location in our department.
   - You may share contact information with fellow members at your own discretion.

2. *Attendance*:
   - First and foremost—*your presence matters!* The degree to which you give and are present in this group is the degree to which you'll receive and learn from it.
   - We certainly understand and appreciate that life circumstances (e.g., illness, fatigue, vacations, family matters) may prevent you from making it to a group meeting.
   - We want to encourage your active involvement in the group (re: group exercises and homework), so that you can get the most out of this learning experience.

3. *Time Limits*:
   - We will be meeting for eight weekly (1.5 hour) sessions, each of which will cover a specific session topic and experiential group exercise.
   - *Your stories matter!* Given this fact, we will be mindful of time, so that each person may be given equal opportunity to share their ideas and experiences with the group.
   - Facilitators will sensitively signal members when it's time to transition.

4. *Personal Meaning*:
   - We recognize that the discussion of meaning is unique to each individual.
   - Meaning may come in *positive* (e.g., life enhancing, loving, caring), as well as *negative* (e.g., anxiety-inducing, sad, disappointing) forms.
   - We ask that the group be open and tolerant of personal experiences of meaning that each member may share.
   - We would like to promote an atmosphere of nonjudgment and understanding, so members may feel free and secure to share their meaningful experiences.

Structured Weekly Topics for Meaning-Centered Group Psychotherapy

Session #1: Concepts and Sources of Meaning

Session #2: Cancer and Meaning

Session #3: Historical Sources of Meaning

Session #4: Historical Sources of Meaning

Session #5: Attitudinal Sources of Meaning

Session #6: Creative Sources of Meaning

Session #7: Experiential Sources of Meaning

Session #8: Transitions (reflection and hopes for future)

INDIVIDUAL MEANING-CENTERED PSYCHOTHERAPY

Inspired by the works of Viktor Frankl, including *Man's Search for Meaning*

Meaning-Centered Psychotherapy Basic Concepts:

1. The Will to meaning: The need to find meaning in human existence is a basic primary motivating force shaping human behavior.

2. Life has meaning: The possibility to create or experience meaning exists throughout our lives, even up to the last moments of life. If we feel life is meaningless, it is not because there is no meaning in our lives, it is because we have become disconnected from meaning.

3. Freedom of Will: We have the freedom to find meaning in our existence and to choose our attitude toward suffering and limitations.

"He who has a why to live for can bear with almost any how."

Sources of Meaning

❖ **Historical Sources** – "Life as a Legacy"
  • Legacy that's been given (past)
  • Legacy one live (present)
  • Legacy one will give (future)
❖ **Attitudinal Sources** – *"Encountering Life's Limitations"*
  • turning personal tragedy into triumph via: the attitude taken toward given circumstances (e.g., physical suffering, personal adversity, one's mortality)
❖ **Creative Sources** – *"Actively Engaging in Life"*
  • via: roles, work, deeds, accomplishments
  • re: courage, commitment and responsibility
❖ **Experimental Sources** – *"Connecting with Life"*
  • via: relationships, beauty, nature, humor

Definitions of Meaning

I. Having a sense that one's life has meaning involves the conviction that one is fulfilling a unique role and purpose in a life that is a gift.

1) *A life that comes with a responsibility to live to one's full potential as a human being.*
2) *In so doing, being able to achieve a sense of peace, contentment, or even transcendence through connectedness with something greater than one's self.*

II. Meaningfulness refers to moments when you feel most alive, connected to existence. Things from the past that, whether tragic or joyful, awesome or dreadful, when you look back on them, you find to be very life affirming and profound.

Meaning-Centered Group Psychotherapy Calendar

Sessions will take place at:

Session #	Date	Time
Session 1		
Session 2		
Session 3		
Session 4		
Session 5		
Session 6		
Session 7		
Session 8		

If for any reason you have to cancel a session, please contact:

Therapist's Assistant/Therapist:

Tel/e-mail:

E-mail:

For other group-related concerns and/or issues, please contact:

Therapist's Assistant/Therapist:

Tel:

Cancer and Meaning

Enhance Meaning
("changing tragedy to triumph")

Cancer ⟶ Suffering ⟶ Find Meaning
(via: sources of meaning)

❖ Physical
❖ Mental
❖ Emotional
❖ Spiritual
❖ Existential

Lose Meaning
("Existential Vacuum")

Homework/Experiential Exercises

Exercise 1.1

(To be completed in session 1)

Meaningful Moments

List one or two experiences or moments when life has felt particularly meaningful to you—whether it sounds powerful or mundane. For example, it could be something that helped get you through a difficult day, or a time when you felt most alive. And say something about it.

_____

_____

_____

_____

_____

_____

_____

_____

_____

_____

_____

_____

_____

_____

Reading: Viktor Frankl's "Man's Search for Meaning"—Part 1

Homework/Experiential Exercise 1.2

Session 2 Preview: Please take some time to think about your answers to the following questions, which will be completed during Session 2 (as experiential exercise for session 2)

Identity before Cancer

1. *Think about a time just before your cancer diagnosis. Write down four answers to the question, "Who am I?" These can be positive or negative, and include personality characteristics, body image, beliefs, things you do, people you know, and so forth. For example, answers might start with, "I am someone who _____," or "I am a _____"*

    Identity after Cancer

2. *Now that you have had a chance to write down some answers to the first question, take a moment to think about how cancer has affected your answers. Are your answers the same? How has cancer affected the things that are most meaningful to you?*

_____

_____

_____

_____

_____

_____

_____

_____

_____

_____

_____

_____

_____

_____

Homework/Experiential Exercise 2.1

Session 3 Preview: Please take time to think about and write down your answers to the following questions to be discussed in Session 3 (as experiential exercise for session 3)
Past Legacy
"Life as a Legacy"
That Has Been Given
When you look back on your life and upbringing, what are the most significant memories, relationships, values, traditions, and so forth, that have made the greatest impact on who you are today? For example: identify specific memories of how you were raised that made a lasting impression (e.g., your relationship with parents, siblings, friends, teachers, etc.). What is the origin of your name? What are some past events or important people that made a meaningful difference in your life? What are the values that have been passed down to you?

_____

_____

_____

_____

_____

_____

_____

_____

_____

_____

_____

_____

_____

_____

_____

_____

Homework/Experiential Exercise 3.1

Session 4 Preview: Please take time to think about and write down your answers to the following questions to be discussed in Session 4 (as experiential exercise for session 4)

Present and Future Legacy

"Life as a Legacy"

That You Live and Will Give

As you reflect on who you are today, what are the meaningful activities, roles, or accomplishments that you are most proud of?

As you look toward the future, what are some of the life lessons you have learned along the way that you would want to pass on to others?

What is the legacy you hope to live and give?

_____

_____

_____

_____

_____

_____

_____

_____

_____

_____

_____

_____

_____

_____

_____

_____

Homework/Experiential Exercise 4.1

Session 5 Preview: Please take time to think about and write down your answers to the following questions to be discussed in Session 5 (as experiential exercise for session 5)

"Encountering Life's Limitations"

1. *What are some of the life limitations, losses, or obstacles have you faced in the past, and how did you respond to or deal with them at the time?*

2. *Since your diagnosis, what are the specific limitations or losses you have faced, and how are you responding to them now? Are you still able to find meaning in your daily life despite your awareness of the limitations and finiteness of life? (If yes, please briefly describe.)*

3. *What would you consider a "good" or "meaningful" death? How can you imagine being remembered by your loved ones? (e.g., what are some of your personal characteristics, the shared memories, or meaningful life events that have made a lasting impression on them?)*

_____

_____

_____

_____

_____

_____

_____

_____

_____

_____

_____

_____

_____

_____

Homework 4.2

"Share Your Legacy"
Tell Your Story

Tell your story to loved one(s) in your life in any manner that is comfortable to you. The key is to highlight experiences that have been sources of pride and meaning for you, or things you wish you had accomplished but have yet to do. As you share your story, start becoming aware of how it feels to have your words witnessed, validated, and affirmed by those who matter most.

_____

_____

_____

_____

_____

_____

_____

_____

_____

_____

_____

_____

_____

_____

_____

_____

_____

Homework 5.1

"Legacy Project"

We want to remind you of the theme "Life as a Legacy" through creating your own "Legacy Project." This is a project that you can undertake that integrates some of the ideas we have already discussed (e.g., meaning, identity, creativity, responsibility, in order to generate a sense of meaning in life despite your illness. Some examples may be: creating a legacy photo album or video, developing a music compilation of meaningful songs, mending a broken relationship, undertaking something you've always wanted to do and have not yet done. . . the legacy is yours to give!

_____

_____

_____

_____

_____

_____

_____

_____

_____

_____

_____

_____

_____

_____

_____

_____

_____

_____

Homework/Experiential Exercise 5.2

Session 6 Preview: Please take time to think about and write down your answers to the following questions to be discussed in Session 6 (as experiential exercise for session 6)

Courage, Creativity, and Responsibility

1. *Living life and being creative requires courage and commitment. Can you think of time(s) in your life when you've been courageous, taken ownership of your life, or made a meaningful commitment to something of value to you?*
2. *Do you feel you've expressed what is most meaningful to you through your life's work and creative activities (e.g., job, parenting, hobbies, causes)?—If so, how?*
3. *What are your responsibilities? Who are you responsible to and for?*
4. *Do you have unfinished business? What tasks have you always wanted to do, but have yet to undertake? What's holding you back from responding to this creative call?*

_____

_____

_____

_____

_____

_____

_____

_____

_____

_____

_____

_____

_____

_____

_____

_____

Homework/Experiential Exercise 6.1

Session 7 Preview: Please take time to think about and write down your answers to the following questions to be discussed in Session 7 (as experiential exercise for session 7)

"Connecting with Life"

List three ways in which you "connect with life" and feel most alive through the experiential sources of:

❖ *Love*

   1) _____

   2) _____

   3) _____

❖ *Beauty*

   1) _____

   2) _____

   3) _____

❖ *Humor*

   1) _____

   2) _____

   3) _____

Homework/Experiential Exercise 7.1

Session 8 Preview: Please take time to think about and write down your answers to the following questions to be discussed in Session 8 (as experiential exercise for session 8)

Questions to think about

Group Experience: Reflection and Feedback

1. What has it been like for you to go through this learning experience over these last eight sessions? Have there been any changes in the way you view your life and cancer experience having been through this process?

_____

_____

_____

_____

_____

2. Do you feel like you have a better understanding of the sources of meaning in life, and are you able to use them in your daily life? If so, how?

_____

_____

_____

_____

_____

3. What are your hopes for the future?

_____

_____

_____

_____

_____

Index

A

antidepressant therapy, *xiii*

assisted suicide, patient requests for, *xiii*

attendance guidelines, *63*

attitudes, choosing, *7, 15, 34*

attitudinal sources, of meaning, *7, 31–37, 66*

attitudinal values, realizing, *10*

authenticity, as a complex concept, *42–43*

authentic sense of self, *16*

B

beauty, *47, 50, 51*

biography, judging, *35*

brain metastases, cognitive deficits due to, xxv

C

cancer

  effects of, *6*

  meaning and, *13–18, 69*

  patients' stories, *9*

  presenting obstacles/limitations, *15*

Cassel, Eric, *34*

check-in. *See* group check-in

co-facilitator model, *xxiv*

co-facilitators

  group led by, *xxiii*

  introducing themselves, *3*

  selecting, *xxiv*

cognitive reframing, *xxviii–xxx*

confidentiality guidelines, *63*

connectedness, to loved ones, *34*

connecting with life, *47, 50, 80*

connection/connectedness, *8*

contemplation, *51*

coping

denial as a method of, *xxv*

  with extreme situations, *35*

  meaning-focused, *xiv–xv*

  optimizing, *xxvi*

  with physical and medical limitations, *36*

core aspects, of identity, *16*

co-therapist model, *xxiv*

co-therapists, group led by, *xxiii*

courage, *42, 43*

The Courage to Be (Tillich), *43*

The Courage to Create (May), *43*

creative and attitudinal sources of meaning, *50*

creative calling, ability to respond to, *42*

creative sources, of meaning, *8, 39–45, 66*

creative values, realizing, *10*

creativity, *42, 43*

Creativity, Courage, and Responsibility theme, *39, 40, 41, 42–44*

D

daily life, finding meaning in, *76*

death

  good or meaningful, *76*

  as ultimate limitation, *7, 15*

demoralization, addressing, *xxiv*

denial, as a coping method, *xxv*

depression, *xiv*

despair

  addressing, *xxiv*

  patients in, *xxv*

diagnosis, identity before and after, *13*

didactic teaching, *xxvi*

discussion, open-ended, *xxvii*

searching for, *6*

significance of, *xiii*

sources of, *7–8*

as a state, *xv*

study's definitions of, *9*

will to, *5, 65*

Meaning-Centered Group Psychotherapy
(MCGP)

described, *xi–xii*

developing, *xii–xiii*

enhancing patients' sense of meaning, *xv*

goal of, *xiii*

overview for therapists, *xxiii–xxxi*

overview of evidence on efficacy of, *xvi–xvii*

randomized controlled trial of, *xvii*

representing the group format of MCP, *xviii*

scientific rational for, *xii*

Meaning Centered Psychotherapy (MCP), *xi*

for advanced cancer patients, *xxiii*

advanced training for workshops in, *xxiv*

basic concepts, *65*

Meaning-Centered Psychotherapy in Cancer, xxiii

meaning-centered statement, final, *58*

meaning-focused coping, *xiv–xv*

meaningfulness, *xxx, 8, 67*

meaningful past experiences, *22*

meaningless, life as, *6, 65*

meaning-making, *xxiii, 5*

members. *See* group members

Memorial Sloan-Kettering Cancer Center, *xviii,
xxiii*

moving walkways, as the transcending escalators,
34–35

mutual learning experience, between all
members, *4*

"my life is my legacy," as acceptable, *57*

N

new beginnings, exploring in and through
Legacy Projects, *57*

Nietzsche, Frankl quoting, *7, 21, 31, 55*

O

open-ended discussion, *xxvii*

outcome assessments, of MCGP, *xvii*

P

painful situations, pride in getting through, *10*

participants. *See* group members; patients

passive appreciation, *10*

passive engagement with life, *50*

past memories, integrating with present accomplishments, *27*

patients. *See also* group members

cancer stories, *9*

definitions of meaning, *9*

excluded from MCGP, *xxv*

selection of, *xxiv–xxvi*

personal experiences, making meaningful, *16*

personal legacy, exploring dimensions of, *23*

personal meaning guidelines, *63*

personal tragedy, transforming into a triumph,
13

philosophy, defined as wisdom of love, *50*

physical actions, defining roles, *16*

physical and medical limitations, coping with,
36

possibility of meaning, from the individual
participant's perspective, *xxxi*

principles, didactic discussion of relevant, *xxvii*

privacy guidelines, *63*

Process Session 1, *14*

Process Session 2, *20*

Process Session 3, *27*

Process Session 4, *33*

Process Session 5, *41*

Process Session 6 and termination, *49*

Process Transition, *56*

prognosis awareness, diverse stages of, *xxvi*

psychological distress. *See* distress

R

real you, being true to, *43*